R00871 92286

DISCARD

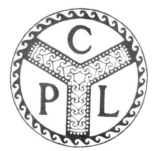

TRIPLEPOINT: In thermodynamics, the state of a pure substance at which *solid*, *liquid* and *vapor* phases all coexist in equilibrium.

— J.H. Keenan

TRIPLEPOINT: In psychotherapy, the state of an individual at which *authority*, *integrity* and *responsibility* all coexist in equilibrium.

— Trevor Trueheart

To

Thea

and all the World's children.

Acknowledgements

I gratefully acknowledge the loving assistance of my friends and colleagues, many of whom cannot be named in this small space. Special thanks. . .

to Carole for teaching me:

𝔊𝔯𝔬𝔴𝔱𝔥 𝔠𝔞𝔫 𝔬𝔫𝔩𝔶 𝔱𝔞𝔨𝔢 𝔭𝔩𝔞𝔠𝔢 𝔦𝔫 𝔞 𝔠𝔩𝔦𝔪𝔞𝔱𝔢 𝔬𝔣 𝔗𝔯𝔲𝔱𝔥;

to Richard B. for the seven league boots;

to Lee S. for providing many keys to understanding,

to Pamela F. for the encouragement surge I felt from her demonstration that text—ink on paper—can heal,

to Laura Walker for hardball proofreading,

to Freda Morris, Elaine Chernoff, and Jens Hansen for penetrating editorial comments, and to all my Tribe brothers and sisters who crossed my path and taught me how to grow.

An Apology

J. Krishnamurti never used the word *I* in any of his many
talks that I attended. If necessary, in responding to a
question from the audience, he would use (sparingly) the
expression, *The Speaker*. He was much wiser than I am.
Of necessity, this book is written in first person; it is the
only way I can share my insight with you. I feel pained by
the repeated occurrence of the name of the **vehicle** of these
experiences when it is the **content** of them which has
importance. It may help you to keep in mind a
metaphysical bumper sticker Alan Watts once published. It
reads:

> *I* am also a *you*!

Table of Contents

Dream content chapters are italicized.

Introduction

Clinical psychotherapy,
esp. drug potentiated

This is how Carole[1] had her specialty listed in the membership roster of the Psychological Association to which she belonged. To her, "drug potentiated" meant, more than anything else, propelled by LSD-25. On several occasions over the years I heard her comment, "The two things that most influenced me were LSD and Aldous Huxley."

Two things which most influenced **me** were LSD and Carole. Over a period of twelve years—bracketing the entire decade of the sixties—I underwent dozens of individual and Tribe[*2] LSD sessions with her. She did not use LSD exclusively; many other drugs were called into use by her. Between the LSD trips, I attended hundreds of

---

[1] Carole Ann Govren, Ph.D. (a pseudonym).

[2] Words marked with an asterisk are defined in the glossary.

"regular" Tribe meetings held at weekly intervals and Saturday night Tribe parties. When I describe this history to people, they universally question the duration of my saga with Carole. Psychotherapy that takes that long has something wrong with it, they say. There were, indeed, things wrong with this therapy, but if I had it to do over again, I would have shortened my time with Carole by perhaps only four years.

During 1961 I attended a symposium where I had the opportunity to meet Dr. Albert Hofman (the discoverer of LSD-25). In response to my question about Carole he claimed her to be a front rank pioneer in the use of LSD in psychotherapy. What better recommendation could there be? Her credentials were solid.

When she first described her Tribe to me, in 1959, she said that these people had all gone beyond the usual goals of psychotherapy. Each had been her patient and had attained the traditional goals. They were, she told me, breaking new ground and going where no one else had gone before in the form of a group. They gathered periodically and collectively consumed LSD. This was her research group. As a university student studying Physics and Engineering with a minor in Psychology, I well knew about research and this description excited me. Carole described the members of her research group as people who were "dedicated to change." So you see, this was presented to me as more than mere psychotherapy.

Carole, bless her heart, required each of us to create a written report of each individual and Tribe session we underwent. In my twelve years with her, I acquired a stack of typewritten therapy papers fully eleven inches tall. These informally drafted documents required much rework and fleshing out. In addition, I have the audio tapes of my early individual LSD sessions, which she meticulously recorded. These cumulatively span a listening period of perhaps one hundred hours. The record is about ninety percent complete; some documents did not survive. The book you are reading was derived from this voluminous material and could not have been written without it.

Another condition was necessary for this writing: It has been eighteen years since I tendered to Carole my letter of resignation from therapy and Tribe. This lapse of time has given me a degree of objectivity about this part of my history I didn't have two decades ago.

Along this arduous and lengthy path, my learning curve remained steep. The experiences I shared with my brothers and sisters in Tribe were painful, awesome, rigorous, exciting, and rewarding. Had they not been, I would not have hung in there as I did. The growth which Carole facilitated in each of us must be acknowledged, and I do so with this book. The trap of personal power she fell into must, I feel, also be acknowledged, because there are others who need to hear this story lest they fall into the same trap. Frequently group leaders, gurus, and cult figureheads have fallen into similar traps. The responsibility and power of one at the top of a human pyramid is too easily corrupted with the growth of this power. It seems to come with the territory and be an inevitable challenge to those who choose the path of power.

Carole demanded that each of her people be "under authority."[*] Yet I had never seen that she, herself, could do this consistently. She seemed to be unable to accept, for long, the authority of anybody else. In her drug work the law required her to have coverage by a medical doctor. In my years with her I watched as she alienated several medical doctors. Many of them (not all, of course) who got close to her work would eventually leave.[3] Either the M.D. would leave her, or she would leave the M.D. In either case, she would often label him or her an "invalid doctor". She was, I believe, absolutely unable to share power. Thus, she would cut herself off from the corrective feedback she needed to remain aligned with the Truth.

This problem, I believe, led Carole to her downfall. She lost a patient under bizarre circumstances which eventually ended her career. Had she not been reluctant to call in the paramedics in a timely manner, she probably could have saved the man's life. She knew, however, that a call to the paramedics would trigger yet another investigation into her ethical behavior and threaten her career. Of course an investigation resulted and the State Board of Examiners ruled that for a period of approximately three hours her patient was in a state of unconsciousness and need of medical attention which she failed to summon during that critical interval. The outcome of it was that the State Board of Examiners withdrew her license to practice.

This, then, is a saga of the sixties—of insights and techniques I acquired during those incredible years. Interspersed with the historical record are selected contemporary dreams I had documented. These round

---

[3] Interestingly, one of the longest of these relationships I watched was with Dr. Adams. During all those years of professional interaction I never saw Carole and Dr. Adams together in the same space. I never saw him attend one of Carole's sessions; in fact the only time I ever saw him was in his office once when he examined my body. The rest of the time his nurse administered everything in his place.

out the activity taking place in my unconscious[4] during my LSD-potentiated psychotherapy.

Will it entertain, amuse, shock you? I hope it gives you some new ways to view your own life experiences and if it should facilitate some healing somewhere along the way then this book will have served its purpose.

How this book is structured

1) Session reports, therapy correspondence and dreams are dated; commentary is not.

2) Dream content is printed in *italics*. Commentary on dreams remains unitalicized.

3) Correspondence quoted verbatim is printed in `Courier`.

4) Fictitious name assignments have grouped family members by initial letter. For example, Charlie is Carol's husband and Chuck is Carol's son. This makes it easier for you to keep track of the characters.

5) Medical Doctors are Dr. George and Dr. Larry.

---

[4] Carl Jung states, in *Dreams, Memories, Reflections*, p348: If the unconscious is anything at all, it must consist of earlier evolutionary stages of our conscious psyche.

In the Beginning

My first marriage was an exercise in tragedy. Soon after leaving active duty in the Navy, I married Terisa, a German nurse I had met a year earlier. She was tall, slender and dignified. We had decided to postpone having children until I achieved my college degree. Tracy was born to us in spite of our taking the care to use a diaphragm. Six months following Tracy's birth, Terisa had exploratory abdominal surgery and was found inoperable with metastasized cancer of the colon. The doctors were shocked that her condition wasn't even suspected until it got that far. The pregnancy had **masked** the cancer symptoms. Her "morning sickness" and constipation were attributed to the pregnancy. The cancer remained hidden until too late. She died two months after the exploratory surgery. I remember telling myself that any time I had from then on was somehow "extra" for me. In my immaturity, I had a notion that I should have gone with Terisa. Our last two months together were not good on any level. Terisa's impending death brought me close to my own mortality. I was scared out of my wits by this confrontation with death, which I could no longer deny. I sealed my feelings off and related to Terisa only on a superficial level. Her final weeks must have felt very lonely.

Later, when my daughter, Tracy, was about two years old, she was diagnosed as being mentally retarded. Her brain, I was told, had been damaged by the adjacent cancer working while she gestated. My life was a shambles. My family cared for Tracy, while I continued with my college studies and part-time job. A year after Terisa died, I met Tammy. In four days we were living together, and forty days after we met, we were married. I fell in love with her independent ways, her long pony tail, her relic of a car, her racing bicycle, and her rebellious nature. We attended the same University. I wanted a woman in my life badly, and we connected something fierce. Her parents were in Europe on a sabbatical leave and she wanted to fill the void left in her life. Tammy, too, was recovering from the bewildering end of a brief marriage, which had been arbitrarily ended by her young husband's parents. Given the degree to which our personalities meshed, it was predictable that before long the dark sides of our psyches would clash. Within our first year, our marriage foundered. In an attempt to salvage it, we sought marriage counseling. Tammy recommended a woman therapist in Stamford—a clinical psychologist—who had helped her work through the residue of an earlier suicide attempt. This person was using an experimental new drug called "LSD". This was in 1959, and I had never heard of this substance. To me, the name consisted of three arbitrary letters. Going purely on trust, I chose to work with this woman, whom I had never met and who used a therapy completely new to me. We would see if we could get our marital problems solved. Tammy and I drove to Stamford and stayed for three weeks in a motel.

During our three week visit, I received three LSD sessions, and Tammy had two. An LSD session with Carole was a full day in duration and was conducted in a private hospital room. As my first session commenced, Carole handed me a small, robin's-egg-blue pill and a glass of water. What I swallowed was 25 millionths of a gram (i.e., 25 micrograms) of LSD-25. I didn't believe that such a minuscule amount of **anything** could impact me. This belief was soon to be shattered as I entered this new phase of my life, which was to endure for over a decade. Two of my favorite descriptions of this path are from Ira Progoff and Marion Pastor:

Although modern psychology began as a medical attempt to heal the sick personality, it is increasingly involved in developing techniques for drawing forth the creative capacity of man. One of the trends in psychology for the past decade has been to explore and emphasize the potentialities of human growth. . . neurosis occurs in the modern world not because of repressed fears but because something creative and meaningful is seeking unsuccessfully to express itself in the life of the individual.[5]

For many years I have been deeply touched and heartened by the courage and love and wisdom—and the capacity for joy and power—that human beings evidence over and over again as they begin to free themselves from the learned belief systems and habitual responses that imprison them. With support and structure, and a framework in which to understand our experience, destructive and neurotic symptoms can fade away as something powerful and real and good within us begins to take over. We are intended for psychological and spiritual growth all of our lives, just as we grow physically when young.

To accelerate your own growth, though, it is necessary to deeply challenge your present behavior, attitudes, and feelings, and your beliefs about yourself, your parents, and your life. In doing this kind of work, either individually or in a group, it is, therefore, most helpful to be guided by a knowledgeable, skillful, and compassionate teacher or therapist who has done the work of healing with his or her own inner child.[6]

---

[5] Progoff, Ira, *The Psychology of Personal Growth*, The Atlantic, Summer, 1961

[6] Paster, Marion, Ph.D., *Anger & Forgiveness; An Approach that Works*, page 177, Jennis Press, 1990.

Carole's Paradigm

Show me a sane man and I will cure him for you.
— Carl Jung

Carole's model of the human psyche, as I saw it, was derived from a blend of many psychological minds and, predominately, from the work of Carl Jung. However, since, in Carole's work, the original trauma must be re-experienced in order to release the patient, she is, to that extent, a Freudian. In Jung's model, there is a conscious mind that you read this with, and there is an unconscious mind which is the domain of both your creativity and your psychopathology. The collective unconscious*, according to Jung, is real and manifests itself throughout your life. Some manifestations of it are quite dangerous.

The unconscious mind speaks to you through dreams, slips of the tongue (or keyboard), drug induced hallucinations, or just plain intuition*. All these channels must be exploited to the full in the service of your growth.

In our correspondence I indicated to Carole that I thought she could speak **directly** to my neurosis. She claimed in a response letter to be able to speak directly to a patient's unconscious mind. It happened often, she wrote, and more often without words than with. This occurred when her patient was under LSD; I have watched her do this with others and had her do this with me during some of my sessions with her. During these times, her piercing eyes resembled those of a hawk.

The unconscious mind is the repository of all your repressions. These are the things about you that are unacceptable to you, so you see to it that, for you in your ego space, they don't exist. Where they go is into your unconscious, where they very much **do** exist. In fact, acting autonomously, from there where you can't see them, they **run** your life. Because you cannot accept them you remain blind to them in yourself. However, when you see somebody else who reminds you of your repressed stuff, you instantly project it onto that person and pre-judge him or her. The **projective** mechanism is perceptual distortion imposed on your world by your own brain. You censor your own data intake to make your world-view conform to whatever reinforces your erroneous conviction that you are not your repressions. Jung called these things, to which you are blind, **autonomous complexes**, and it is maladaptive (and neurotic[*]) to let them run you. Your repressions must, in therapy, be brought to surface consciousness one at a time, like peeling layers off an onion. You can expect to cry some with each layer, also like peeling an onion! With each repressed incident in your life, there is a residue of highly charged emotion. As the repressed material surfaces in dream images or LSD sessions (through hallucinatory sensations that feel absolutely real), these emotions must, if you are to grow, be accepted, and fully felt.[7] They must be acknowledged, expressed and discharged, no matter how fearful or abhorrent they make you feel.

---

[7] Albert Hofman, *LSD, My Problem Child*, 1983, pages 48-9:
Another significant, psychotherapeutically valuable characteristic of LSD inebriation is the tendency of long forgotten or suppressed contents of experience to appear again in consciousness. Traumatic events, which are sought in psychoanalysis, may then become accessible to psychotherapeutic treatment. This does not involve an ordinary recollection, but rather a true reliving.

This psychotherapeutic paradigm is not held by all. R.D.
Laing claims that "The way in (meaning the path you took
to your present neurotic condition) is not the way out." He
pioneered alternative directions in psychotherapy to
prevailing concepts based on psychoanalysis. However,
Carole's method worked well with me.

Imagine you are part of Carole's Tribe. As your repressed
material finally surfaces to consciousness, now within the
safe space created by Carole, the emotional energy that you
have carried all through life, since the original incident,
may now be released. You should have expressed it back
then, but, to the detriment of your mental and emotional
health, you did not, often because its expression was either
forbidden or perceived as life-threatening. Now, as you re-
experience the emotional reality of your original incident,
as you are regressed back to its time and it becomes
contemporary with your present ego consciousness, now is
your opportunity to safely express this emotional charge.
This is your abreaction. At last, for you, Carole has
created a safe space for this to happen. Now is the time
for you to scream your rage or choke on your sobs. Tribe
members are called upon to stand in for people in your
past: siblings, parents, uncles, teachers, or whatever is your
need. The original scene is pretend re-created but your
reality is **there** back in the original event. History can now
be rewritten. This time you have the opportunity to express
the forbidden emotions. You may yell, scream, blubber,
spit, insult, threaten, and do just about anything you want
in expressing the residue of emotional charge in the repression, except you cannot physically injure yourself, or
anyone else. The context of Tribe has provided you with a
safe space to do this. You are sheltered, supported,
encouraged—and sometimes commanded—to encounter
something that has secretly (or otherwise) terrified you for
years. Only by engaging and accepting your fear, as it

comes into your consciousness, may you free yourself from continuing to carry this psychic load. After all, it takes psychic energy to keep it hidden and to reshape your world impressions until they don't threaten your belief system. Otherwise, you will be troubled by inconsistencies between what you see and what you believe.

Almost always, part of the repression consists of feelings of guilt. Carole labeled this "past-time" guilt. It is unleashed with the liberation of the repression. Present-time guilt, on the other hand, is created when you fail to fulfill obligations, day-to-day duties, and that which Carole called *framework*. This was one of Carole's most-used tools of psychotherapy. It is the label she used for those activities one must do to get through life productively and guilt-free. This could include paying one's bills on time, meeting one's obligations and commitments, and, in general, meeting the challenges of life in a responsible manner. Any framework break will result in present-time guilt, which acts like a magnet hooking into your past-time guilt from a repressed incident. Thus present-time guilt can act as a valve opener to your past-time repressed guilt. You can feel swamped in all this guilt, which is out of proportion to your present-time framework break. With this kind of aperture* into your personal past-time guilt you expose yourself to, in addition to your own repressed energy, pathos from the collective unconscious mind. This situation demands "asepsis*" and maintenance of each and every piece of your framework.

The *stash-dump* period evolved out of necessity. Our Tribe sessions too often focused upon mundane daily conflict of one kind or another. Resolving to cope with these petty demands of relationship before we got into the Tribe drug experience led to the ritual of stash-dump. Sometimes this took many **hours** at the beginning of a Tribe session. This began the session during which we each spoke to anything that might get in the way of the session, such as emotional baggage for another or completing something left incomplete in a relationship. No one could attend a drug session with either a load of guilt or a pending emotionally charged issue with another person who was present at the session.

The path to creativity is to free your unconscious of these repressions that run you and whose unconscious energy you must constantly supply. To free yourself from your repressions, one by one, you must gather hints about their content and correlate this material with conscious knowledge about your past. Then a creative leap or insight must occur.

Once, at one of my LSD therapy sessions, I had regressed back to a very early age. Kurt, a long-standing member of Carole's research Tribe, and a New York TV director, was in attendance. He and Carole were trying to figure out why I had been chewing on my lower lip during the session. Being in this state, regressed in consciousness to a very young age, I was unable to comprehend what they were talking about and so couldn't enlighten them about it. Kurt closed his eyes, wrinkled his face like he was squinting hard, as though to see something through a fog, and reported imagery he received that came out of **my** repressed past:

You are about four years old. You have a fuzzy, pussy-willow-thing which you put into your nose. It gets pushed in tight. You can't get it back out. You call your grandmother for help. She can't get it out either. She takes you to a doctor to have it removed. The doctor takes you into his clinic and lays you down on his examination table. He has one of those round mirror things on his forehead. After removing the pussy willow from your nostril he reaches down and fondles your penis. Then he leans over to kiss you. At this you bite him, viciously, on the lower lip.

(This incident is further elaborated in a later chapter.)
My conscious mind replied that my doctor then was one
James Little. Did he do that to me? I had always
remembered him as being gentle and kindly; my memory of
Dr. Little didn't track with this image.

Months after this session, when I was next with my mother,
I asked her about the pussy willow thing in my nose. She
replied that once, when my parents were out and my
grandmother was watching out for me, this had happened.
She had no transportation to get me to Dr. Little so she
walked me to a doctor she knew about, who was only a
few blocks away. Nobody in the family knew anything
about this doctor, and this was the only time I ever saw
him. So Kurt's vision of my own past history was cor-
roborated by my mother. Evidently no one in my family
ever knew about this doctor's attempt to sexually molest
me. Only I and this doctor knew that I had bitten his lip,
and I had repressed the incident until it surfaced in Carole's
therapy.

I have no explanation for how it was that Kurt could
perceive a drama that I carried, buried, in **my** brain.
Clearly, we have facilities we don't know of and little
understand. Later, at the Catskill Halloween session, I did
exactly the same thing. I 'channeled' a dramatic scene
from the unconscious mind of each of two Tribe people in
rapid succession. This, also, is more fully discussed later
in this book. My understanding of this phenomenon
remains void; it lies outside of cause and effect. To simply
label something as *ESP* does nothing to aid understanding.
If Carole can "speak directly to the unconscious," of
another then why is it not possible for some of us to "see

directly into the unconscious" of another?" John Lilly observes that,

Whether something is perceived as 'hallucination' or as receiving (psychic) communication from another (i.e., telepathy) depends upon one's belief system, so choose whatever interpretation you wish.[8]

In addition to being the source of your creativity and the vessel of your personal repressions, your unconscious mind, according to Carole's paradigm, may carry an "It." This is an unnameable entity living in your mind, as a tapeworm might live in your gut. Typically it entered you during childhood when you were under anesthesia in surgery, under a high fever, or when you were knocked unconscious in a traumatic accident. These are among the things to be expelled by exorcism[*], which occasionally took place during Carole's Tribe LSD sessions.

Carl Jung[9] describes the process this way:

page 187:
The essential thing is to differentiate oneself from these unconsciousness contents by personifying them and at the same time to bring them into relationship with consciousness.

page 192:
. . . I took great care to try to understand every single image, every item of my psychic inventory, and to classify them scientifically—so far as this was possible—and, above all, to realize them in actual life. That is what we usually neglect to do. We allow the images to rise up, and maybe we wonder about them, but that is all. We do not take the trouble to

---

[8] John Lilly, *John Lilly, so far*, p86

[9] Jung, Carl; *Dreams, Memories, Reflections*

understand them, let alone draw ethical conclusions from them. This
short-stopping conjures up the negative effects of the unconscious. . . .
Insight into them must be converted into an ethical obligation. Not to do
so is to fall prey to the power principle, and this produces dangerous
effects which are destructive not only to others but even to the knower.
The images of the unconscious place a great responsibility upon a man.
Failure to understand them, or shirking of ethical responsibility, deprives
him of his wholeness and imposes a painful fragmentariness on his life.

This also explains why some people have "bad trips" on
LSD. If one takes this drug to be merely entertained by the
images produced, then instead of meeting the
responsibilities they bring, one meets the negative effects of
his unconscious.

Following my years in psychotherapy I conclude there are
three reasons for pursuing this difficult life-path: 1) To
enlarge ones repertoire of choices in life, 2) To fill the
voids in ones education left unfilled by earlier training and
teachers, and, 3) To resolve and release inner conflict.
Since **anybody** can benefit from more choices (which is
what freedom is all about), and has **some** holes in his
education, then competently conducted psychotherapy
would be of universal benefit. Why our voting populace
shuns any political candidate who has psychotherapy in his
history puzzles me. After all, he may be the only candidate
whose sanity has been certified.

Ira Progoff offers a vivid description of the excitement I
felt on being joyfully swept away by Carole's therapy:
The reactivation of the natural process of growth is accomplished
primarily by learning to participate more fully and harmoniously in the
continuing flow of imagery which is the main content of the psychic
processes. The term "imagery" as used here refers not only to visual

imagery but to the flow of all kinds of non-conscious phenomena- words, intimations perceived within dreams, and so on. From this perspective, the job of psychologist is to draw the flow of the psyche onward, to generate an ever greater momentum of psychic activity. The feeling of an interior momentum is a feeling of meaningful life welling up within the individual. When the individual begins to experience the reality of this interior flow, he has achieved the essential contact and has gained access to the larger sources of the stream of life energy.[10]

---

[10] Progoff, Ira, op. cit.

On the Safe Release of Rage

Writing this book is a wonderful experience! Daily I mentally review what I have written and gathered. Always I wonder, what comes next? Always I feel that I will come up short of content. And always, the writing for that day floods out in a deluge.

This morning it was triggered by a radio interview I heard. The woman interviewed was an incest victim who was discussing her healing, her many modalities of therapy she put herself through. She struggled to get complete, in her consciousness, to accept the reality of her early abuse with inner peace, and to get on with life. She spoke of a core of unconscious anger she had been, and still was, carrying and how she learned to discharge some of it. I immediately place her situation in the paradigm of Tribe dynamics. She spoke of her difficulty in reaching forgiveness. I judge her path as leaning too heavily toward forgiveness when, until the hostile energy is released, forgiveness is moot.

If anything ran through the core of Carole's belief system about her patients (not to mention the world at large) it was their repressed **hostile** feelings and how to confront them.[11] This was where Carole shined. She was a master

---

[11] *Anger* is a feeling resulting from mistreatment or injury. *Rage* ia a furious, uncontrolled anger. *Hostility* is a feeling of enmity or desire to hurt.

Carole almost universally used the word *hostility* instead of the others. *Anger* and *rage* both derive from being hurt by another. *Hostility*, the desire to do harm, is qualitatively different. I feel that *rage* would have been more appropriate in

at catalyzing anger and its expression. She created a **usually** bullet-proof psychic wall at the boundary of physical violence. She taught us about this wall and all its loopholes. Anyone who attempts to bring on rage in the service of therapy and of the creative, must know how to keep it physically safe. Carole's principle tool was the **commitment.** To watch it in action was astounding. The set of words which evolved out was simple:

> Today, I, Trevor, will not physically
> injure any person.

Before a hostility discharge session (or *any* therapy session) was commenced the set and setting was highly structured. The dischargee had to say the above sentence flawlessly. Sometimes this took twenty seconds, sometimes it took twenty minutes! The number of permutations and combinations of ways to alter the above simple sentence were astonishing. Great creativity was displayed in verbal loophole attempts. People new at stating this commitment started by simply not retaining it all in short-term memory. After three or four attempts it was in memory, then the dance began! The wrong name would come out. The word "physically" would be omitted and the person would sincerely believe it had not. Sometimes a word was added, resulting in ". . any *other* person." Thus, the self was omitted from the commitment, etc.

Carole's work, which might be described as uncontrolled internal anger whose outward expression is controlled by circumstances set up by her. That Carole chose, instead, the word *hostility* reveals an orientation to the world that I do not share.

Occasionally the wall would not hold. At the Coaticook session[12] Ned, a somewhat schizophrenic man who enraged easily, threw a Pepsi bottle and a flower pot at Carole. As a result he spent the night tied, hand and foot, to a lawn chair.

From all appearances one would believe that Carole had a double standard of behavior. She could slap someone across the cheek but no one else could. She could resort to hurtful physical contact but no one else had that privilege. On a few occasions this issue was discussed. The slapping was to make someone move through their stubborn resistance to seeing and consequently to changing. Carole described her need for slapping patients: it was to abort or prevent violent behaviour and sometimes to bring hysterical patients into reality.

Brought to question was, "Who among us is now consistently clear enough to use slapping creatively instead of as an expression of his/her own repressed hostility?" Guilt was the contaminator. With guilt, one's perception is distorted and reality-picture not to be trusted. It took particular clarity of soul, a pure being, not to abuse this borderline act of violence. Two or three of the most "maturely evolved" of the Tribe were seen to be clear enough for this duty sometimes but not consistently. Thereafter it remained Carole only who could slap. She used this act infrequently.

---

[12] This session was held just over the Canadian border at a rented building on a small rural "fat farm" fitness ranch. This was to remove our drug activity from U.S. jurisdiction.

Marion Pastor clearly describes the valid and invalid expressions of anger:[13]

page 82:

"Anger is the only alternative children have to placating or going numb when they feel punished or abandoned by their parents."

"From the beginning, our anger is usually either falsified or repressed. False anger is anger that is directed at the wrong target, in the wrong moment, or for the wrong reasons. It blinds us to reality and perspective. False anger strengthens the "I'm right, you're wrong" syndrome, forcing us to see the target (often ourselves) as wrong and evil. Repressed anger is a poison, and causes us enormous stress.   Furthermore, repressed anger always "leaks out" in some way to spoil our relationships with other people and with our selves.

page 81:

"Anger is an almost indispensable tool in arousing strength we need to break out of the beliefs about ourselves and the world that we learned when we were children.   Unleashed, righteous anger, directed specifically against the mental images that keep us fearful, inadequate, unloving, and unloved, can work magic in freeing us to affirm our real selves."

pages 127-8:

"...anger is always a way of handling fear. As long as we remain angry, we are still afraid. It is not possible to feel real compassion for someone we fear."

"If we stay angry, we must hold on to pain, fear and resentment to justify our anger, which means that we continue to live with pain, fear, and resentment.

page 130:

"If we cannot reach compassion within ourselves, we are caught in believing that the only way to be strong is to be tough and angry. The reality is that the stronger we become, the safer we feel, and the more tender we can be.

---

[13] Pastor, Marion, PhD, ibid.

These truths about anger from Dr. Pastor reveal the value of Carole's approach. In my own case, my childhood expressions of anger toward my parents were not only forbidden, they were unthinkable. My father, a reserve military officer, was not disposed to have anyone "talk back to him". Any expression of anger was viewed as insubordination. His children were no different from his enlisted men in this respect. My anger, unexpressed, left me numb to my feelings. More than anything else, Carole worked to bring my feelings to consciousness where I could take responsibility for them. Carole released her patients from the fear underlying their anger by challenging them to scream their righteous anger at the limiting mental images they carried.

However, Carole had her people perpetually screaming at one another. When I left her therapy, group meetings were routinely begun, as they had been for years, with five minutes of each person present screaming at others present, whether they needed it or not. The breakthrough to compassion, described by Pastor, never seemed to occur. It is my belief that Carole herself never broke through to lasting compassion.

Hatred and hostility is a mode of life accepted by many people in the western world as the normal way of doing things. As a chosen lifestyle, however, it is very stressful. Bhudda said you will not be punished **for** your anger; you will be punished **by** your anger.

You find yourself living with that anger, hatred and bitterness, all that stuff that comes out of you in the name of getting someone else to change, or not liking the way the world is, or expecting the world to be the way you want it to be instead of admiring and celebrating the way it is. You get punished by your anger that you live with all of the time. It intensifies your life-stress, makes your heart beat faster, raises your blood pressure and creates all kinds of physical maladies. Expression of rage during therapy has some limited use; as a lifestyle, no thanks.

Carole's non-violence commitment is deeply engraved in my memory. To this day, I use it often. Before I start up my chainsaw, climb a ladder, or initiate some other hazardous activity I pause for a moment and run the commitment words through my consciousness. Doing this forces me to examine things closely and see what must not be neglected to insure my safety. Occasionally, as I do this, I choose to postpone the activity completely until I give more thought to what does not feel right about it.

Alpha Box; My First LSD Session

My first interview with Carole was on 24 June, 1959. The next day I had my first LSD.

Tammy and I had come to her in hope of salvaging our marriage on which many—particularly Tammy's parents—had already given up. We were each very neurotic and our neuroses were interlocking and hopelessly entangled. We cheated, stole, lied, and generally sabotaged one another's efforts. Furthermore we each thought the other was acting out of malice when, in fact, it was more like just plain neglect and selfishness. We had no idea of what we were into, much less how to get out of it.[14]

Tammy's parents, Tina and Tomas, were appalled to learn that their daughter had married someone she had met only forty days prior and whom they had never met or been told much about; they were both in England on sabbatical leave

---

[14] This mistaking of neglect for malice, by the way, happens frequently whenever communication breaks down. The most dramatic example imaginable of this changed the consciousness of virtually everybody! It is described by Paul Simon in his *The Tongue-Tied American: Confronting the Foreign Language Crisis* (New York: Saber Press-Continuum, 1980):
"What millions of Americans remember most vividly about Nikita Khrushchev's historic bridge-building visit to he U.S. back in 1955 is his belligerent promise:

"We will bury you!" Yet he never said it. What we heard was a translator's version of the Russian expression, "We will *outlive* you!" Whatever the realities of Soviet political intentions, all the top Russian meant to assert on that occasion was the superiority of his system over ours.

during this period. Predictably, within our first year together, our marriage foundered. Tina and Tomas considered me a basket case. Tomas, a professor of organic chemistry at the University, knew Carole through a shared professional interest in LSD. They were instrumental in sending Tammy and me off to Carole, in Stamford, for three weeks of marriage counseling a lá LSD-potentiated psychotherapy.

Carole was taken aback, upon meeting me, at the wide disparity between how she saw me and how Tammy's parents had described me. She had expected to meet a monster. Tina and Tomas had shaken their heads, washed their hands, and given up on the marriage. Carole was startled with pleasure when I walked into her office and she saw, not a monster, but a man with the hands of a farmer and the head of a poet, looking like a young monk from an early Botticelli. However, as soon as I attempted to speak she saw my difficulty. I was almost completely nonverbal as I attempted to describe my feelings to her. Intuition is one of my greatest innate strengths but my parents didn't knowingly operate from or even much acknowledge the existence of intuition. To speak my mind I had to strain words through the layers of intuition and sort them out with my logical mind that had been, as Carole described, "hooked up by an artistic prankster." My difficulty was compounded by the fact that my logical mind had not been, until then, introduced to the existence of my intuitive mind.

During our three week visit in Stamford, Tammy and I stayed in a motel room. Following my first office visit with Carole she had me obtain a general physical examination to clear my way for receiving LSD.

The doctor who examined me completed his work-up by writing, on one of his prescription blanks:

To Dr. Govern:
Mr. Trevor Trueheart is in good shape;
OK for LSD.

I hand-carried this back to Carole who inserted it into the file she kept on me. Curiously, the prescription was not dated.

This document cleared my way to receiving three day-long LSD sessions, and Tammy received two sessions, all during these three weeks. These took place in a hospital room. A medical resident at the hospital, Doctor D., was available as medical back-up for Carole.

Set and Setting
In her experience, Carole had learned some extremely effective techniques in doing therapy with her patients. Music was used extensively in every drug session whether individual or tribe. She had collected a repertoire of pieces which have provocative effects in facilitating work with unconscious material. She sat in a chair beside the bed on which I lay. Next to her were a tape recorder, microphone, note pad, and L.P. phonograph. The music she chose might be a Sibelius symphony or a Chopin piano concerto or something from Wagner. Over my eyes I placed a black cloth mask to block out room light and lay relaxed on the bed while Carole played a side of music. I was instructed to "go with the music and otherwise just **be** with what happens." When the music finished I was to remove the mask, bring my consciousness back into the room and tell Carole what I experienced. Describing the imagery—mostly visual and in color—but sometimes kinesthetic, tactile, auditory or olfactory, Carole would become interpreter for me. She heard my symbology of these dream-like images and responded by telling me how

they were meaningful in my life-dynamics. For example, the mistletoe leaves and berries I hallucinated were symbolic of the integration of the male and female aspects of my psyche. These, growing together on the same plant were growing in coexistence. The sharp edges on the (male) leaves and the bitterness of the (female) berries revealed my inner lack of harmony with regard to both my sexual identity and how I related to others.

Creating life changes

Toward the session's end, and at subsequent meetings, Carole and I would discuss what therapeutic **changes** to effect in my life. These were then instituted into my daily routines. They represented our response to the messages contained in the material produced by my unconscious mind which had emerged during the session.

My soul was greatly troubled at this beginning of my psychotherapy. My frustrations, guilt feelings, conflicts and lack of both self-esteem and self-confidence gave me endless material to work on during the session. With Carole's capable assistance I began the long, long process of sorting them out, understanding them and instituting life-changes.

That evening, after I had become quite fatigued from the day's work, I wanted to stop the struggle with myself that had gone on that day. However, I was unable to stop the steady stream of conflicting feelings and images that came into my consciousness. I was listening to some soft meditational music and trying to rest peacefully but found that a thousand and one of my old, worn-out images were swimming around in front of me. Most of them reflected either hostility or conflict. I had stopped going after them, seeking them out, and was now trying to avoid them, not because I was afraid of them but because I was damned tired of looking at them. Enough for one day! With the need to disconnect from the heavy work of therapy I then found (invented? discovered?) my BOX. Tired, and in a twilight near-sleep state, I found myself, in my imagination, withdrawing into a small box. The walls were good, solid, break-proof glass held in a stainless steel frame. It was cubical in shape, four or five feet on a side and just large enough to hold me comfortably. The sides, front, and top were hinged so that I could reach out and pull them shut forming a closed box. There were rubber gaskets along the seams effectively sealing me in. Inside this imaginary closed box I discovered I was no longer bothered by the images that had been swimming in my vision. They remained out there, outside the box, and I could still see them if I looked, but now **I didn't have to look at them if I didn't want to.** Inside this box I found the peace and freedom from whatever part of me had been hammering at me with all the images.[15]

Within the week following a session I wrote up my session report. These were typewritten and typically two or three pages long. Carole read the report, noted items to discuss with me later, and filed it.

I kept a carbon for myself that I also filed. Carole wrote her own report on my session, of course, as she did with all her patients. Most chapters in this book began as session reports, originally written twenty-five or so years ago and recently rewritten and edited for consistency and completeness. Simply re-working and completing this material has been a therapeutic experience for me.

------

[15] Since this session I looked for this box on occasion but it was not to be found. It was not until my final LSD session twelve years later that it reappeared as OMEGA box. Then it was not a box where I found peace and freedom but the opposite; it felt like a restraining cage to me.

The LSD sessions had their timing, their rhythm. Usually, a month or more elapsed between them. This was because it took that long to integrate what was learned, from this experience, into one's daily life. The unconscious material elicited during a session were expressions of discontent. (After I had worked through my repressions my unconscious energy of discontent, upon its release, turned into creativity). These expressions of discontent had to be interpreted and acted upon. The messages were translated into life-changes and these changes had to become a part of my new life. This process of integration took time as I changed habit patterns and took on new and different activities, duties, commitments, and responsibilities.

Unconscious material from "Freudian slips" (either spoken or written) and from dreams were just as useful as that released by LSD. These insights appeared on a daily basis. My dreams would often **continue** work on an issue begun (but not completed) at an LSD session. Alternatively, and with full symmetry, some of my LSD sessions began by continuing work triggered by an earlier dream. I might bring to a session a typewritten description of a puzzling and troubling dream—of a few nights prior—for Carole to read. Under the LSD, however, when I was reminded of the dream its meaning often became so immediately obvious to me that I wondered how I could have been so dense as not to see it earlier. Both my conscious and unconscious mind were immersed in—and thriving on—the therapeutic process.

Carole's principle working tool for her patients[*] was **framework.** The life-changes were **framed** and might consist of abstaining from shoplifting, getting a book chapter written by a certain date, washing dishes after meals, or whatever seemed most needed by the patient. Any breaks in one's framework were brought up at meetings and discussed. The patient's resistance to therapy was reflected by his or her framework breaks. Of course an overdue therapy payment was always a framework break!

The ultimate goal was to **achieve** as one moved through life. Neurotic hangups got in the way of achievement and had to be confronted and abandoned. Achievement, for an individual, might be professional advancement, acquiring a university degree, getting a book published, or producing a child. As each person's potential was unique so were his or her achievement goals. This work required a highly structured lifestyle. Framework meant commitment of one's time and energy toward certain goals. It brought focus and intent to bear on the achievement goal.

On Dreams and Dreaming

If a man devotes himself to the instructions of his own
unconscious, it can bestow the gift, that suddenly life,
which has been stale and dull,
turns into a rich, unending inner adventure,
full of creative possibilities.

— M.L. von Franz, *Man and His Symbols*

Very early in my therapy I began writing my dreams, daily,
in a journal. As I did this, over the months, I found that I
was writing more and more dream content each day. My
ability to recall minute detail increased with practice. After
about two years of this I found that I was writing dreams
for nearly two hours each day. That got to be too much
and I cut back dream writing to only those which had a
high impact on me. This I have been doing ever since and
I typically document a dozen or two dreams a year.

Writing this, as I enter my sixth decade, I look back and
see that there have been very definite themes to many of
my dreams. An example is when I quit tobacco, after a
thirteen-year addiction. My earlier four failed attempts to
quit taught me that the critical event for me was that very
first puff of a cigarette. During these efforts I learned that
I had convinced myself that I could have just one hit of
tobacco and then successfully back off to abstinence. I
learned this was self-delusion. If I could just hold stead-
fastly against that first puff I would succeed. If ever I
yielded to that first intake then I knew the whole edifice
would come tumbling down and I would be back to a pack-

a-day within a month. So what recurring dreams did my unconscious give me?

After my long addiction to tobacco smoking and four failed attempts to quit, both my conscious and unconscious mind lacked confidence that I could overcome my addiction. This was revealed by this recurring dream:

I found myself with a short burning cigarette in my hand. I had just become aware of it and of my surroundings. Worse, I felt sick to my stomach as I realized that I had just smoked half of it unconsciously! I had crossed the critical threshold with no conscious awareness of doing so. Consciousness of the event came after it was too late. My decision making capacity was out of the loop at the critical time. I felt sick with the realization that I knew what was coming: being once again conquered by my tobacco addiction.

What purpose did these recurring dreams serve in my life? They kept me humble; they kept me from getting too cocky and daring about tobacco. They served to remind me that I dare not demonstrate I had overcome its influence by, for example, inhaling just once at a party to show off to my friends how I could "control my addiction."

For two months after I stopped smoking, I had phy-siological withdrawal symptoms. During this time I would actually reach out my hand toward the cigarettes that were no longer there. For two **years** I had psychological withdrawal symptoms. During this time, whenever I was under stress, my mind would reach out toward the nicotine no longer there. The body speaks to the mind. When the body is addicted to tobacco it can speak with great urgency.

Another recurring dream lasted for **exactly** six years. Korea was our war when I enlisted into the navy. My "agreement" with Uncle was to serve two years on active duty and six more years on "inactive reserve" status. That meant that if there were another war during that interval Congress could call me back to active duty. Upon my transition from active duty to civilian life I thought about the remainder of my agreement very little—if at all. I was in nearly complete denial that anything would happen to require my return to the Navy. My unconscious mind didn't deny it at all. Hell, it created my return to the military over and over in my dreams. I would find myself in a barracks, in uniform, suddenly comprehending the fact that I had been "re-enlisted." It was a horrible nightmare and at the end of the six years, following my final discharge, I never had another one like it.

Carl Jung taught us that dreams serve a compensatory function. In this case I was experiencing fear and anxiety in my dream life that I was refusing to confront consciously.

Dream Chemistry

If you are interested in your dreams you might consider making a Mugwort pillow.[16] Mugwort is an herb and grows as a weed where I live. Gather a few handfuls of Mugwort leaves. Dry and crush them and sew them into a pillow, then sleep on it. If your experience is like mine you will have quite vivid and astonishing dreams.

Pearson and Shaw[17] suggest vitamin B-12:

This vitamin can cause spectacular intensification of colors in dreams or sometimes even produce colors in dreams of people who never before had colored dreams! It works about half the time in the small group of people we know who have tried it. (Sometimes the colors are so vivid they can

---

[16] Jeanne Rose, *Herbs & Things*, Grosset & Dunlap, 1972, page 149

[17] Durk Pearson & Sandy Shaw, *Life Extension*, 1982, page 195

wake you up!) A dose of one thousand micrograms or so is effective.
Take it **just** as you get into bed to sleep."

Also, try exploring **lucid** dreams, in which you become
aware that you are, in fact, in a dream. The book *Lucid
Dreaming*[18] explains how it is done. In a nutshell, here is
the technique: You wake in the early morning with a recalled dream. Examine the dream in your mind until you
are in good contact with the feel of it. Next imagine yourself back in the dream but this time with the knowledge
that it is a dream. Then say to yourself that you will go
back to sleep and re-enter the same dream knowing you are
dreaming. If you then go back to sleep you are likely to
have a lucid dream, but not necessarily a continuation of
the earlier one.

As I mentioned, dreams are one of the doorways to your
unconscious but it is not **just** another doorway. The
advantage of dream study is that you dream every single
night. Each day of your life your unconscious offers a
message for you. June Singer[19] reveals this when she
writes,

The whole point of dream analysis is to teach the patient eventually to
become independent of the therapist, by acquiring the ability to carry on
the dialogue with his own inner aspect which has a therapeutic quality,
that is, with "the therapist within."

---

[18] Stephen LaBerge, Ph.D, *Lucid Dreaming*, 1985

[19] Singer, June; *Boundaries of the Soul*; page 276, Doubleday.

Commitment to the Truth
Tribe Seed Session of 10-6-62

"Cogito ergo sum"

I think, therefore I am, as put forth by Descartes, presupposed **thought** as a condition of existence. After this seed session I am convinced that "I **feel,** therefore I am." My feelings, as a result of this session, have become a sufficient condition of existence and more convincing to me than my thoughts.

There were eight Tribe members plus Carole present; this was the smallest Tribe session I have yet attended. I took six capsules of seeds[20] and one spansule*®

---

[20] These were capsules of Morning Glory (Ipomious Tricolor) seeds ground up in a coffee grinder and put up in capsules. I had purchased *two pounds* of these seeds from a large seed company (one pound for Carole the other for me) shortly before word got to the seed people that this species seed offered more to people than pretty flowers. Richard Evans Schultes, in *Hallucinogens of Plant Origin* in *Science*, Jan., 17, 1969, (as reported in *Licit & Illicit Drugs*, The Consumer's Union Report on Narcotics, 1972, page 345), writes:

"For many years chemists sought to isolate the active principle in these morning-glory seeds without success. Since 1960, the mystery has been solved. The hallucinogenic seeds contain a chemical very closely related to LSD. Most of the morning-glory seeds available in the United States, however, are believed to lack both this drug and the LSD-like effect."

My experience differs. I know I would be unable to distinguish between the effects of 100 micrograms of LSD-25 and 100 morning glory seeds. I have heard, among other rumors, that such seeds are now treated to make them unfit for human consumption.

of dexedrine® (a member of the amphetamine family, or "speed")

The first half of the session now seems hazy to me. The Tribe began by lying, prone, in a circle with heads toward the center. Theme for the session: proceed toward his or her personal Hell. I didn't feel much movement. I felt I should "allow myself to descend" with no active pushing on my part. I thought I might arrive in Hell by simply dropping my psychic barriers and passively allowing myself to be taken there. Never did I feel I had a definite procedure for going to Hell. Carole commented that, curiously, Hell felt **cold** to her rather than hot.

The Tribe changed position; we sat facing the center of the circle. There was no agenda and what happened did so spontaneously. Our new position brought me a memory of a football huddle of long ago. Carole, who sat at my right, was expending a lot of energy in hard psychic work for, I thought, someone in the Tribe. I could tell this from her breathing, feeling her heartbeat through her hand, and the feeling of energy passing through our hands. Then I realized that I, too, was an energy channel and my energy was going out my right arm and into Carole. Looking around I could see all others appearing to be going through something similar. As I watched this I saw that the work occurred in pulsations. Collectively people pushed through a lot of effort and then stopped to recover their strength or draw in energy to replace what had just become depleted.

Later the rhythm changed into a push-pull mode between Carole and me. It was as though she would "push" or "lift" something and then, having temporarily exhausted herself, draw back, whereupon I would pick up the action and "hold" whatever it was so it didn't slip back, during which time Carole gathered more strength. Then, just as I felt about exhausted from holding the thing she would come back and pick up the load and lift some more while I, in turn, recovered from the effort.

I remember a strong smell during this activity. I couldn't tell if it was physical (objectively in the room), or my hallucination, but it was a strong odor of shit. I thought that somebody must be having foul-smelling poison pushed out of his body.

The seeds were peaking at this time and I felt out of it. It felt possible that I was one of the people being psychically worked on by the Tribe. During the earlier huddle and seemingly connected with the effort I was now expending, my left arm began quivering. Later on this was to become significant to me. Perhaps the intense work I had been doing was releasing a repression in me. There are so many possibilities I'm not sure what happened at that time.[21]

The next event was a period of relaxing and lying around with most people enjoying the **feelings** of love and sexuality. As always during our Tribe sessions, this took place without any **acting out** of sexual feelings. Carole was teaching us to discriminate between genital sex and the a-genital feelings of sexual flow that can occur between two non-penetrating people. Curiously, we felt this flow more in the solar plexus than the genitalia. I was lying on the floor next to Ollie, my electronics buddy who shared a lot of interests with me. Kurt was lying in a human puddle with Don and Debbie. This couple, Don and Debbie, were a tower of strength when together. They had five kids who were all active in Tribe affairs. Kurt began to display his

---

[21] It was not until decades later that I gained an understanding of why the body quivers, buzzes, or vibrates during an emotional release induced by a psychedelic drug. It represents the tissue response to liberation from chronic control.

sexual feelings in a visible way. To use Tammy's term, he was "dry fucking," that is, humping while fully clothed. I watched this out of the corner of my eye and felt anger toward him. Why I felt this I wasn't sure. It had something to do with his overtness in showing his sexual feelings. About this time my left arm began quivering movements again. Kurt got up and lay next to Carole. I felt more angry as I watched him. Then I thought I must have felt jealous of his freedom to feel sexuality but now I think it was connected with some exploratory homosexual incident from my childhood. I had not been allowing any of **my** sexual feelings toward Ollie to come to consciousness while Kurt had just enjoyed his sex feelings with two women in the Tribe. I realized that all this I felt was my own baggage from my past and, in reality, had nothing to do with Kurt.

Everybody except Ollie and I then got up and went into the kitchen to get food. Ollie and I remained because of the emotional stuff I was yet experiencing, and Ollie stayed to assist me. I believed that I had to allow my feelings of sexuality for a man (Ollie) up to consciousness if I was to get to the problem I had with my anger toward Kurt. Several times I could feel the sexuality begin to come into awareness but it had a strange quality. I would feel a sensation of intense, physical, sensual feeling at the very tip of my penis. As soon as I would feel this my left arm would quiver again. I realized I was strongly defended against allowing the sexual feeling and was fighting it. After several minutes of this I realized no progress was being made. Ollie asked me what I wanted to do. For a few minutes I thought about it. Intuitively, I got that it was really Kurt toward whom I must feel the sexual attraction since I instinctively knew that, on a deep level, Kurt and I were sexually attracted to each other. I didn't know if I could go through the experience of allowing my sexual feelings for Kurt with just him and me, or whether I would need the support of the rest of Tribe to do this. Also, I didn't know if I **wanted** to do this at all. At the time it would have been easy for me to just drop the issue and not deal with it at all. As I pondered this I realized that **this** was the moment for which I had been working so hard in therapy.

Weeks prior I had a strange feeling about the hard, daily swimming I had been doing to get my body in good condition. I had felt that I was preparing myself for some impending battle. Suddenly I knew that this repressed memory I was working out **was** the battle I had been preparing myself for. Also, I knew that this moment was the point in time at which all the conditions were fulfilled for going through with it: The Tribe was there; Carole and her strength were there; Kurt, the one most likely to catalyze the thing in me was there; we were at a session whose purpose was to help individual growth. Everything was perfect. The stage was set. So I was faced with the ultimate question: Did I really **want** to grow? The question couldn't be avoided. This was my supreme moment of truth. I made my decision, got up, and walked into the dining room and asked Kurt and Tribe to come help me.

At this part of the session the concept of "commitment to the truth" took on a crucial meaning for me. I could easily have avoided the whole issue at the time I first felt the anger toward Kurt with its accompanying veiled psychic threat. For me, "commitment to the truth" meant nothing more than "look at the facts." It had nothing to do with the courage to either evaluate the facts or go ask for assistance. Commitment to the truth didn't mean "go through a painful experience," it simply meant "look at what is." I didn't fear looking at the truth except that if I did, I might then have no option but to move toward that which I **really** feared, that which lay buried in my unconscious. I could have looked at a slightly different mindset of facts and concluded, validly, that I wasn't ready to deal with the repression. As I sat on the floor, wondering what to do, I could feel the presence of the defense, the neurosis, almost tangibly. I even told Ollie I could feel it. My way out, in the past, had been passive resistance and procrastination. This had something to do with commitment to the truth. These modes of resistance say, "dump it for now . . . do it tomorrow . . . or better still, never." In my past I had always made some identification with this time-stopping resistance. I used it to avoid pain at that instant in time. Now, I am getting a clear picture of this mechanism—even as I write this report—and I now see into the part of the resistance I could never identify or own. Now I see that I had been equating the **avoidance of pain** with the act of **avoiding the facts**, the truth. This is a pattern of behavior which had been reinforced again and again until eventually I believed that the two are really connected in some way. Hence I adopted this as my means of defence against pain which is a kind of denial. I was afraid of fear itself. Now I know that there is no connection between the two. Facts are facts.

As it turned out, once I had made the decision to ask for help, I found that nothing which followed was painful. Had I not made that move I know now that the remainder of the session for me would have been a kind of slimy, death-like, **painful** event. In fact, the remainder of the session was productive, rewarding, and happy. The outcome was just the opposite of what I anticipated.

As I write this, events of the session take on new meaning. When I remember Don burying his head like an ostrich I think of my passive resistance which is the same class of behavior. When I recall Kurt speaking of fearing that I might break his back I think of how I felt the moment I decided to ask for help. I was struggling with something which felt alien. It turned out to be my own resistance and at that point in time, when I made my decision to get help and confront this, I "broke the back of the neurosis."

Again, as I write this, I feel like I am going through another session. Again and again, insights come to me and many minute memories of the session come back to mind.

As I began writing this I was trying to describe something about the neurosis and the identification factor. There must have been a **strong** misperception at work. I had been equating burying my head with the absence of pain. In reality, my avoidance of the facts—of the truth—had been the **cause** of most of my psychic pain. Now I know that pain does not lie in openness to the truth so my aversion to looking at the truth is beginning to lift.

Carole, Kurt and the rest of Tribe came into the living room. Kurt and I sat facing one another and we locked eyes. Then I could watch clear imagery of what had happened to me and I described what I encountered. It had been a repressed memory of events which took place when I was three years old. My family, eking out a living during the depression, lived in a small rural cabin on a farm. Beside our cabin was a corn field. It was summer and I was wandering through the corn stalks which towered over me and concealed me from view from the cabin. I had to urinate which I tried to hold in. Spontaneously my penis grew erect. An older neighbor boy came by, perhaps attracted by my erection. He fondled it until I came (my first time) whereupon I lost control of my bladder and sprayed the boy with my piss. The sexual feelings I had were new, confusing and intense. I was emotionally open and psychically vulnerable. I expected the boy to act lovingly toward me but instead he beat me up for peeing on him. In my confused openness I became a receptacle for the boy's sexual guilt, sexual inadequacy, and anger. As he beat me up he pounded on my left arm and so hurt it that it quivered for the next hour or so.

During the session, as my arm underwent this quivering I said that it felt like my arm was "possessed" by something. In hindsight, it is no wonder I felt such fear going into this. It was a coming to consciousness of a fusion between my first sexual experience and immediate and painful violence to my body. I had made the incorrect conclusion that a sexual orgasm felt, at first, incredibly good then was immediately followed with painful punishment. The memory of the pain in my arm certainly came forth in the session as the twitching. Until I allowed its re-creation, with Kurt standing in for the older boy in the cornfield, the memory in my head was inaccessible to me.

Dr. Pastor addresses my experience precisely:[22]

. . .it is often when we stand up to what frightens or enrages us—when we allow our experience to deepen and find the strength to go through it—that our lives are most rich.

Had I chosen to cop out and not confront my facts I know that I would be walking an alternative path in life, a much more neurotic one.

---

[22] Paster, Marion; op. cit., page 163

Therapeutic Dreamwork
12-5-62

In rapid succession I had the following four dreams

First dream:
I was walking through a large city with heavy traffic. There were many irresponsible drivers who would run through red lights, drive excessively fast, etc. I had to be careful in two ways: 1), I had to obey the traffic laws myself, and 2), I had to watch out for the many others who did not themselves obey the laws. It was not sufficient that I have my framework together; I also had to stay aware of the invalid acts of others in order to survive.

The conclusion, that I must be doubly vigilant in life, certainly applies to one undergoing the self-examination of psychotherapy.

Second dream:
I was watching an old wooden house which was on fire. There were firemen there and they put out the fire but not until most of the house had been burned up. The house had been full of combustibles and trash. The refuse of the family who had lived there had accumulated, for years, in the house. The house was drab, rundown, and grimy. Two children who had lived there were killed in the flames of the fire, while a third child, in the confusion, had wandered out into the snow. She was never seen again.

The house, run down and full of the trash of years, represented **me,** I reflected. The two children lost in the flames were the two abortions I had induced and the child

lost in the snow is Tracy, my mentally retarded daughter.
The firemen were the forces of the life situation which led
me to therapy and the growth process.

Third dream:

*I was viewing a pleasant scene in nature. It might have been
part of a park. There were rolling hills and terraces.
However, this land was covered totally with rocks, all about
the size of a softball. They were several feet deep on the
land. The firemen from the second dream appeared and they
picked up the rocks and hauled them away to the city dump.
They left the land in its natural condition, as it had been
before people covered it with their rocks. There was one
difference. If the rocks had never been there the land would
have been covered with grass and wild flowers. I knew that
these would now begin to grow on the land. There were a
few rocks remaining but these belonged. They were partly
imbedded into the soil unlike the rest which were simply
resting on top. As the last fireman was leaving I said to him,
"Not a stone out of place."*

Here, **the land** is what I identify with. The rocks represent
the accumulation of psychic loads[*] I have picked up from
others over time. In the presence of these loads the grass
and flowers could not naturally grow. The rocks partially
buried represent my own legitimate loads and
responsibilities in life which I must carry. These rocks had
a beauty about them and reminded me of a cultivated rock
garden or landscape. They were part of the natural beauty
and did not impede the plant growth.

Fourth dream:

*The scene was a lake with a pier which led out over the
water. I stood on one of the pilings and, hanging on my back
with arms around my neck, was a small boy. I jumped off the
piling and began to fly over the water at a fairly low altitude.
I was showing the boy what it was like to fly. After a while*

we flew back to the piling and landed. Then some adults came nearby and I started to tell them about this mode of flying but they seemed skeptical about the possibility. I told them I thought everybody had the potential to fly. One asked me, if they had the potential to fly, then why couldn't they? I told him that they would misuse the gift of flying so that, for them, it remained only potential. Wanting to demonstrate to them my flying, I saw another small boy, about the size of the first one, and told him to climb on and we would fly together. In order to let him climb on I squatted down. As he climbed on I was astonished at his great weight even though he was no larger than the first boy. He was so heavy I could hardly hold him. The strain of holding him as he climbed on my back was so great that the seat of my pants split down the seam. I stood up with great effort. I didn't know if I could fly with all this weight but I decided to try. I jumped off the piling and we began to fall but we descended slowly since I was carrying as much weight as possible with my "flying mechanism." We landed in the water but didn't sink very far because I was still "flying" or at least carrying some of the weight. I began to swim toward a ladder some thirty feet away. About halfway to the ladder I felt exhausted and stopped efforting to carry the weight. We both sank deeper into the water and I continued to swim to the ladder. As we swam I looked at him and said, "Boy, you are really loaded." Then he said I couldn't fly after all. I pointed out that I had carried half his load during the first part of the swim, the truth of which he had to admit.

This dream had a positive quality since I had chosen to fly under safe and appropriate conditions for all concerned. In flying low over water nobody would get hurt if I crashed. The results of my work in therapy, symbolized by dream flying, were beginning to free me from my neurotic obsessions.

As I lay in bed, awake, thinking about these four dreams, I felt good about them; each had felt rewarding. Then I pondered about the one thing that didn't seem to have meaning. Everything seemed to have an "obvious" interpretation except for the splitting of my pants. I thought about my childhood when I had been coerced to submit to anal intercourse by some of the older boys in the neighborhood. Immediately one older boy came to mind. I felt that the dream resulted from a sexual load I had picked up from him during the anal incident. Perhaps this is why I had been mixed up about sexual and bowel loads ever since. I had carried this boy's sexual load in my bowels where he left it. After working out this notion I got up and went to the toilet to try and unload this thing. All that I could produce was flatulence but as I did I visualized imagery of blowing out the psychic load I had carried since childhood. My body felt lighter and began to tingle with new feeling. Again and again, my therapy consisted of getting in touch with my feelings, and I was learning to use any bodily discharge efficiently in the service of my growth.

The boys I flew with were aspects of myself, of course. (In a real sense, **all** creatures in dreams represent some aspect of the dreamer.) One was encumbered with psychic loads and I sank with him and his load. With the first boy, unencumbered, I easily flew. The message is clear. This is what my psyche is getting out of therapy.

Behind the Looking Glass
LSD session of 2-8-63

"O Aswins, lords of Brightness,
anoint me with the honey of the bee,
that I may speak forceful speech among men."
— the Atharva-Veda

In a private room at a small Connecticut coastal hospital I took 150 micrograms of the free-form of LSD on this day. This was the strongest single dose I have had. It was a new formulation and felt about one and three-quarter times as strong as the tartrate form of LSD.[23]

While waiting for the drug to take hold, Carole and I discussed some of my dreams. When I was only four years old I had awakened one morning and proudly announced to my parents that I had dreamed I learned the alphabet. I

---

[23] There is nothing static in drug research. Albert Hofmann, in *LSD, My Problem Child*, 1983, page 31, writes:

"When a new type of active compound is discovered in pharmaceutical-chemical research, whether by isolation from a plant drug or from animal organs, or through synthetic production as in the case of LSD, then the chemist attempts, through alterations in its molecular structure, to produce new compounds with similar, perhaps improved activity, or with other valuable properties. We call this process a *chemical modification* of this type of active substance. . . . Many LSD derivatives were produced since 1945."

Some of the LSD I had consumed were such newly isolated derivatives which came from laboratories at north eastern universities.

then boggled both their minds by flawlessly rattling it off to them without pause.

A more recent dream placed me with my first wife, Terisa, who had died of cancer. I was saying goodby to her. At this part of the session I wanted to approach her death and when I did I broke into tears. I did this several times and each time Carole told me that I had nothing to do with her death. She said that she has completed her circle and mine was only half done. I had some confusion at this time about whether I was alive.

The drug came on quite rapidly and I soon transcended the dimension of **time.**

The session seemed alphabet oriented, starting with the alphabet dream. Now there appeared a "B" or "bee." I heard the buzzing of a bee and asked Carole what one does if one discovers a bee which has flown into one's clothing. I felt that the thing to do was to slap the area where the bee was felt and kill it before it could sting. What this symbol meant I'm still not sure. The buzzing of the bee, which I clearly heard, was an auditory hallucination. As time s—t—r—e—t—c—h—e—d out for me, the buzzing noise slowed down to a series of statico repetitive sounds that were somehow like the individual pictures on a strip of motion picture film. This kind of stopping time felt artificial; I thought time should have been transcended instead of stopped. It represented a kind of freezing or solidifying process and felt like I was close to the core of the neurotic process. The sound then changed from a slowed-down bee to a helicopter. Have you ever listened closely to the sound of a helicopter?

I speculate the frequency of this noise drives certain brain waves to have the effect it does on me.[24]

I don't know if the bee thing is good or bad, desirable or not; I don't feel a strong identification with it. I do feel that if one goes into a cosmic plane of existence—and goes with the grace of God—that it should be a smooth, letting-go-of-gravity process instead of the pounding statico of the helicopter buzz. This was one time my unconscious expressed itself in therapeutic growth without my conscious understanding of what happened.

Kurt came into the room and I held his and Carole's hands in my own and a very strange thing happened. The buzzing of the bee/helicopter grew very strong in my head. My back arched, I tipped my head back until my mouth pointed at the ceiling. Then I grew rigid and my mouth opened wide and the bee/helicopter flew out of me and went straight upward. I felt it move up from my navel, ascend through my throat and mouth and leave my body. As it left, some part of my psyche ascended to the cosmic level of being.

The rest of the session was most strange to me. I had always pictured the human psyche as divided into a conscious part and an unconscious part with a surface in between these two like the mirror in Alice's looking glass. Normally, dreams and other unconscious material are dark, foggy or otherwise obscured from direct vision. I receive the unconscious material symbolically perhaps because they come from a part of my brain where logic and words are absent. These communications must be spontaneously created by my unconscious mind and expressed in cryptic,

---

[24] *Alpha* waves in the human brain fall in the range of 8 to 13 Hz. I estimate helicopter sounds run in the 20 to 30 Hz. range, which corresponds to *Beta* waves.

symbolic hints. When I think about it I feel astonished at how much my dream mind must **create** to tell me something. During the session I found myself on the **other side** of the mirror. I could see two obscure, filmy people near me (Carole and Kurt) but could not communicate with them for they were now on the other side from me.

My memories of recent events in my life, such as the drive down to this session, running out of gas, picking Tammy up at the airport, and last night's party, became unreal and dark as though it were **these** events that were dreams. I lost hold of conscious reality. If it became dream-like to me and the world of actual dreams solid and substantial, then what and where was reality? The world became fluid and structureless and I could find nothing **invariant** that I could use as a kind of anchor. I tried speaking. I struggled to utter the word, "reality"—as if I could contact it if only I could speak the word—but I couldn't find the apparatus for speaking the word. I was in the midst of one world and I was unable to communicate with those in their world on the other side.

The filmy barrier—the mirror between worlds—shifted. It appeared on Carole's face; the mirror's plane split it vertically. The right side (Carole's right) appeared to be a reflection of the left side. Later my whole field of vision appeared split, vertically, into two halves, one a mirror image of the other. My rational mind had the notion that it should have been split horizontally, like looking at the surface of a still lake, but it wasn't. The curious state I entered is elsewhere described by Carl Jung[25]:

When the libido leaves the upper world of light, whether by individual decision, or owing to the decline of vital energy, it sinks back into its own

---

[25] Jung, Carl, *Symbols of Transformation*, 1956, Princeton University Press

depths, into the source from which it once flowed out, and returns to the point of cleavage, the navel, through which it once entered the body. This point of cleavage is called the "mother," for it is from her that the source of the libido came to us. Therefore, when there is any great work to be done, from which the weak human being shrinks, doubting his own strength, his libido streams back to that source—and that is the dangerous moment, the moment of decision between destruction and new life. If the libido remains caught in the wonderland of the inner world, the human being becomes a mere shadow in the upper world: he is no better than a dead man or a seriously ill one. But if the libido succeeds in tearing itself free and struggling up to the upper world again, then a miracle occurs, for this descent to the underworld has been a rejuvenation for the libido, and from its apparent death a new fruitfulness has awakened.

I remember being asked, by Carole, if I wanted a shot of Ritalin®*. She had to ask several times, clearly and loudly, to reach me. I struggled to comprehend her question and managed to utter the word *yes*. It wasn't the conscious "I" that knew I wanted it. It was some part of my unconscious, my intuitive source, that decided for me. My conscious mind couldn't even understand the question; I had never had IV ritalin before and so had no reference with which to evaluate the question. The nurse in attendance at the hospital ward was Mrs. B. At first I had assumed that her only role was that of duty nurse. I was surprised to become aware of a deep closeness I felt toward her. She came across like a Tribe member—one of "the family." I felt I had known her a long time. As she injected the twenty milligrams of Ritalin into my vein I could feel—quite distinctly—a vast amount of psychic strength coming into my arm. The shot must have been my personal miracle for it filled me with what I needed to break through the wall of my hung up libido.

Carole and Kurt each took my hands. Then I was able to really let go to the drug and regress to where I felt like a

mentally retarded child. I couldn't speak or even voice
words. Carole spent two hours teaching me the alphabet.
Later she told me that I had taken a shortcut by learning it
in my childhood dream. I had to be taught the alphabet at
age twenty-eight because I had ducked the task when four
years old. The struggle to learn my ABC's in that hospital
room was very real.

Mythology literature yields, as usual, food for thought[26]:

The bee represents mother-matter as a vessel of transformation, from
which honey, the golden spiritual food, and mead, the liquor of inspiration,
are born. And both of these lead naturally "from mouth to breath, and
from breath to word, the logos." As such an alchemical vessel, it bestows
the gift of poetry, an art which clothes in musical word-form the fleeting
shapes and smells and sounds of outer nature, the feelings and the images
of the inner world.

---

[26] Gerry, Peggy, *Reflections on the Symbolism of the Bee*, lecture delivered
to the Analytic Psychology Club of Los Angeles, April, 1961.

Parenting: A Critical Issue

A central rift zone in our marriage was the issue of offspring. Tammy thought she wanted to have a child; I did not, at least not yet. After our first few years of marriage she began to feel her biological time clock running out, while I maintained that we were not yet emotionally mature enough to be parents. The longer we waited the more urgent this grew for her.

Here was a "catch-22" situation for us. The longer the clock ticked the more urgent Tammy felt about conceiving. The more urgent she felt about it, the more she leaned on me to impregnate her. The more she leaned on me—to do that which I felt we were not ready to do—the more I resisted her pressure. And, finally, the more resistance I put up, the more strife came between us. So, instead of growing toward parenthood in therapy, we instead found ourselves growing further apart over the very issue that was supposed to cement our marriage.

During my first brief marriage, Terisa and I had decided to defer creating children until we reached certain vocational goals. Tracy came to us unexpectedly in spite of our careful planning and efforts. Shortly following Tracy's birth I lost my wife to cancer. Not long after that I lost my child, to mental retardation, as she failed to develop normally.

Carole, following her clinical paradigm, was convinced that I carried some repression that was blocking me from being open to the joy of parenting. During several of my LSD sessions she searched for this repression, believing that, upon bringing it to the light of day, I would be released into fatherhood. Carole "knew" that I had, buried somewhere in my mind, a "reason" for my resistance. This repression could be reached with the aid of LSD. Actually it took **two** sessions. The first one was when she told me, over and over, "Terisa's cycle is complete, yours is only half complete." The second was when I had become, in my drugged state, a woman who had just given birth to a child. Carole had "delivered it" and she joyfully held aloft the baby, which was her discovery that my resistance had been springing from my unconscious belief that if I had another child I would lose it. This would be a replay of my earlier tragedy with Tracy. She assured me that my wires were crossed. The pounding I had taken over Terisa's death and Tracy's mental retardation was not the universe's way of saying I will lose my future children. "That doesn't apply anymore," Carole explained. She told me, "You now have a strong, healthy body, a strong healthy wife, and a strong healthy Tribe matrix to help you all the way. Now is the time for you to go with the incredible creativity that comes with rearing a child."

This interpretation of Carole's never rang true to me and I maintained my resistance to assuming parenthood. In truth I wanted children in my life someday but my strong conviction remained that neither Tammy nor I were then capable of undertaking this responsibility. I stated as much, repeatedly, to both Tammy and Carole. People, saw enormous potential for creativity in my relationship with Tammy. The whole Tribe seemed to be cheering us on throughout these early years at Stamford. Everybody wanted us to have a child including me. Where I differed from everybody else was simply in the timing. My position was that, if Tammy and I could not yet successfully manage our own affairs in relationship, then how could it be possible for us to do justice to rearing an infant? I wanted to hold off until both Tammy and I learned how to work together in loving cooperation instead of our continuing pattern of mutual sabotage. It was clear to everyone that we had not attained that level of functioning together. All too often, we gave each other enmity instead of emotional support. This was not, to me, healthy ground on which to rear a child.

When Carole "uncovered" my secret resistance, she announced it to everybody, and declared it null and void. Therefore I should now be free to go forward into parenthood. Inside, I didn't feel much had changed except that any future expression of resistance I might utter would now be declared invalid. If I still said that I didn't feel ready yet, I was told to discount that feeling. The reason for this was that **nobody,** I was told by all, **ever** feels ready. And, since my "huge unconscious block" had been excised by Carole, why was I still holding out?[27]

During a vacation trip to Canada in 1963, Tammy and I made love in a motel room. When I withdrew before ejaculation Tammy broke into tears over my doing so. I am an incorrigible sentimentalist; I simply cannot tolerate my loved one crying. That, combined with a feeling that we were making reasonable progress in therapy and

---

[27] Contrary advise is rare but it does exist. Kelsey and Grant write, in *Many Lifetimes*, page 201:

"There is no reason whatever why a couple should feel obliged to have a child. There are already too many people in the world, and if there is a genius waiting to come in, there will never be a shortage of fertilized ova from which he can choose. In developing their relationship with one another a couple may well be doing all that in this particular lifetime they have set out to do; and a couple who radiate happiness are an asset to the community of incalculable value."

therefore our future would, hopefully, be secure, I relented and impregnated Tammy the following night. In doing so I questioned my judgement and took a chance anyway.

Now everyone in Tribe, our brothers and sisters, seemed to be awaiting the blessed event. They, and Carole, were so much a part of this creation that Thea, our new offspring, was universally viewed as a "Tribe child."[28] The common view was that Carole and Tribe had salvaged an extremely creative union and the issue of that union, Thea, was the pride of all. Tragically, this would prove to be Thea's burden as well.

---

[28] Thea was not the only Tribe child; the youngest child of Debbie and Don was also born into the Tribe environment and was viewed as one.

Dreams Keep Me Honest
Dream of 6-4-63

In a letter to Carole I described my efforts to obtain a new job. The personnel manager at Smyth Instruments, where I had been laid off, told me that until my accrued vacation period had run out I could tell people who interviewed me that I was still on Smyth Instruments' payroll. Technically, this was the truth; however, I told one interviewer, "You can reach me at Smyth Instrument Company," which was no longer true. My description to Carole included the following dream:

I was watching a scene which consisted of several men with submachine guns who were shooting at a stained-glass window. The window appeared in brilliant colors and was round and large with a mandala-type pattern. The men were a group of revolutionaries, a lá Castro, bearded and dressed in army fatigues. All of them were firing at the window and the panes were rapidly being shot out.

Here it would seem that the forces of chaos and destruction were destroying the spiritual element. The meaning of the dream seemed obvious to me in connection with the job interview, so the following Monday I drove back to Cambridge and went to see the interviewer and told him that I had misrepresented myself and the actual position I was in. It didn't seem to make much difference to him but it sure did to me. I didn't look forward to telling him and correcting his awareness but I knew it had to be done. Once done I could feel a load lifting from my shoulders. I found subsequent interviews much easier and I was able to

express myself more freely and with an enthusiasm I didn't
have with the preceding ones.

My statement to the interviewer was clearly a borderline
case—a half-truth—until I was led into an out-and-out lie
and then I had to backtrack to restore my integrity. It also
was clearly a case of violating part of my framework
(commitment to the truth), but I restructured it by returning
to the scene and lifted the guilt from myself by the seemingly painful process of confessing to the man that I had
lied. We live and learn. I now know, from this, that I
can't state even a half-truth and get by my unconscious
with it.

In the same letter to Carole was another dream:
*I was on the campus of MIT, and I was talking with one of
the professors. Along came a man on horseback. I felt
identified with and empathetic toward this man, who reminded
me of Don Quixote. The hooves of the horse were very thick
and untrimmed, as though the horse had not received proper
care. The man was carrying a ladder on his shoulder. He
put the ladder down on the ground and rode off. Next, seven
or eight men from a rival campus (Harvard?) came walking
toward the professor and me. They were looking for some
kind of mischief. They didn't concern me because I didn't
consider myself part of their rivalry battle. They saw the
ladder, picked it up, and started to carry it away. This
disturbed me since the ladder was somehow connected with
me and I suddenly became involved. I spoke up to them and
said, "Not the ladder!" I walked over to them to engage
them. They dropped the ladder and picked me up, some on
my arms and some on my legs. I was held horizontally, face
upward. They began to pull me in all directions as though to
tear me apart. Some kind of power battle was being fought
between these men and me. In spite of the disproportionate
numbers I felt the balance of power to be about even. This
was because they were using only physical power on me and*

I had a kind of psychic power available to me that they did not have. I called upon God to give me the strength to do battle with these people. I spoke to some unseen entity I knew was with me, saying "OK, let's drive it under!" This referred to some collective possession which was inciting them, and this I had to drive underground.

Up to that point I felt no fear or terror because of the confidence and help I knew I was receiving from the unseen entity. The struggle had taken place for some time and when I said, "OK let's drive it under," something became triggered and I underwent a psychic transformation. Something took hold of my mind and body and I went into convulsions. At the same time I watched the overcast sky above me boiling with turbulence. As the convulsions started, a hole appeared in the cloud layer. It got larger and larger as the convulsions grew. Through this hole I saw an unbelievable blinding light. Perhaps it was this fantastic brilliance that caused the convulsions. With each convulsion I made a loud grunt actually issued verbally and these woke both Tammy and me. As I watched the hole open up, the clouds around the hole's perimeter were violently swirling. I knew this meant strong anger connected with the source of the overwhelming light. I had a feeling of impending "doomsday" and thought the light on the other side of the cloud layer would destroy everything.[29]

After I woke up I had no feeling of dissociation which I might have expected. I knew I had been dreaming and I

---

[29] This doomsday feeling is adequately described by Whitmont in *The Symbolic Quest*, 1969, page 292 (G.P. Putnam's Sons, NY):

"A great many people who think they live in fear of the atom bomb are in reality afraid of a psychic atom bomb—the compressed power of unknown inner needs which are vaguely sensed as a threat that might shatter the seeming peace which the conscious adaptation has established."

knew that I had just awakened and I knew where I was. I lay there with closed eyes and could still see the receding light. I pondered the meaning of the dream for a few minutes and began to feel psychically loaded in connection with its content. I got up in the darkened room to go urinate the load out. While I felt no residue of fear carried over from the dream I did want to feel something familiar. Jurgen, my German shepherd dog, walked over to me. I buried my hands in his warm fur for a long moment. He felt wonderful and I thought it not unlike the grounding I experience when I immerse my hands in a container of water. Finally I entered the bathroom, urinated and visualized the psychic load flowing out my body in the stream of urine. It felt complete; the load, whatever it was, was dumped.

The way my body was held immobile, by seven or eight men in this dream, resembled the process of Carole/Tribe doing a physical *mummification**. The resulting overwhelming experience certainly was congruent with Carole's mummification goal. That goal is to induce psychic change and movement through one's resistance to growth or through one's attachment to the neurosis. The clinical psychologist's definition of *God* is "anything that is overwhelming."[30] If being held to witness a light grow to universal destruction (starting with me) is overwhelming, then it could be said that in this dream I had encountered my maker.

In this dream everything was rational until the horse and rider appeared. I was completely familiar with the campus after many years there as both student and employee so the scene could easily have been a slice of my waking life.

---

[30] Spoken by Dr. Marie Louis von Franz in documentary film *The Way of the Dream.*

The man on horseback was myself, muddling through life like Don Quixote from one bizarre scene to another. The neglected hooves reflected my patchwork sense of responsibility and the ladder represented, to me, my chosen path of LSD depth therapy and climb to wholeness. He put the ladder down and I felt protective of it as I highly valued what my psychotherapy was accomplishing. In my struggle to protect this life-path I found myself overwhelmed and confronting Armageddon. My path to growth, maturity and creativity would be, evidently, an overwhelming one. I couldn't figure out whether my unconscious was making me a promise or a threat, but somehow I felt good about the dream.

Positive States of the LSD Experience
"Special Methedrine®"[31] Session of 11-30-63

The weeks immediately preceding the session were hard for me. Tammy and I were not communicating and I found myself living with a lot of pain and grief. On top of that, the events surrounding the John Kennedy assassination impacted me on both personal and collective levels. Through all of this I held firm to my framework and remained surprisingly operative and in touch with my feelings, however negative they had been.

The session opened with everyone taking fifteen milligrams of "special methedrine" except for Tammy, who, being pregnant with Thea, of course took none, and I, who was in need of getting "unhooked" (mostly from my emotional dependance on Tammy) took thirty milligrams. So this time it was I who took the point position. Like several previous Tribe sessions, one person had a high dose and the rest small doses of *booster*[32].

---

[31] "Special methedrine®" was a code expression signifying methedrine (a member of the amphetamine family, or "speed") tablets onto which an accurately measured amount of liquid LSD had been deposited (i.e., pipetted) and allowed to dry. Thus two drugs are swallowed in one tablet although usually only one of the two was mentioned.

[32] A term which I coined in 1963 for the purpose of disguising our language. Initially used as a synonym for LSD it later signified *any* psychoactive drug. There was a period when clinical use of LSD, while not yet rendered illegal by the government, was a hot issue among both researchers and clinicians using it. To

The first hours (in fact it seems for most of the session time) were spent with the Tribe members sitting in a circle expressing whatever reservations they felt about anyone or anything. As this took place I felt the special methedrine take hold and entered a state-of-being as rewarding as it is rare.

Let me generalize the positive states of the LSD experience which seem to fall into two categories. There are those which open my being to **relationships** on the deeper psychic levels and those which open my psyche to the cosmic. The first deals with relationships with other people, the second with relationship or communion with God. While there is no real difference between these, i.e., the presence of God is most strongly felt through the acceptance of, and the bonds with, other people, there does seem to be a distinction on the operational or experiential level. I am describing two facets of the same thing. The people/relationship facet is characterized by a down-to-earth stream of various sensations and events. Things and feelings are perceived directly. There is an acute awareness of my body and its sensations and feelings. On the other hand, the cosmic facet may be described by an almost complete removal of the "flow" of things and an entrance into the "eternal now" at which point there is no motion as is ordinarily known and no sensation as is commonly felt. Instead there is the awareness of the presence of the "blinding light," to use a phrase from Tibetan Buddhism. This has been my most direct and powerful experience of the presence of God. It has always been accompanied by a feeling of uncertainty that I would survive the experience because of its very intensity.

---

avoid criticism we elected to keep a low profile on our activities.

During the early part of the session, stash-dump time, I entered a state that does not seem to fit either of these descriptions. My state had some of the best parts of both and some which neither of the experiences described above have. The first thing I felt was the effect of the special methedrine acting like 'psychic lubricant'. Slowly—but quite definitely—all the events of the preceding weeks took on meaning and significance which I hadn't felt before. I felt myself becoming "the perceiver." I was not the objective, disdainful, withdrawn perceiver as stereotyped scientist. I felt very much a part of what was happening and deeply a part of the relationships which were both complicated and involved. I, as perceiver, was able to see, directly, what felt like the complete reality of all of the complicated relationships.

Several times through the day, I perceived the session, people and events to exist in a medieval setting. The Tribe seemed to be having the session in a stone castle. Carole, dressed in black and wearing a large circular pendant, appeared to be a combination of a page boy and Merlin. While these are both male figures the reality of the situation seemed beyond sexual identity. Carole, very much a woman, had many of the characteristics of these males from past time. What is the "reality" of my perception? In our quest for growth our Tribe must be doing what has been done before and I felt a bond with the other people who have gone through these experiences in the Middle Ages.

As I watched Ollie talking, dumping his stash, I, the perceiver, saw him as the equivalent of a piece of stone. He was something that someone had carved and chipped from granite. After much talk Ollie took his special methedrine and his stone-like aspect melted away. I was astounded at how strongly and directly I had been **seeing** his resistance and how I felt that it blinded him. The contrast between him and me seemed severe in our respective ability to perceive at that time.

As I watched the events unfold, many of the faces and other parts of people and parts of the room took on the appearance of a Picasso painting. Parts of faces and objects seemed to shift and take on an angularity. Was I seeing things in their primal forms? As I felt my perception get sharper I saw faces and objects "go double" as one sees a "ghost" on a TV screen. Seeing double was a transition state my psyche was passing through. During another transition state some of the faces took on the appearance of being smeared, as one would smudge a still-wet oil painting of a face by wiping a hand across it. The smear was always horizontal and appeared only on faces, not on objects. Also, I saw it only on some but not all of the faces. The smear and double visions did not have the feeling of being aberrations or distortions. They just appeared and did not disturb me. I made no effort to "focus" these effects away but instead found myself fascinated by this manner of seeing things. (When I am resistant to seeing something my tendency is to passively make things go out of focus, which I have to fight consciously. This mundane, neurotic, visual distortion is totally different from what I now describe.)

After I went through the transition states I felt in complete accord with the reality of the session and it was this state which I value most of any I have ever experienced with or without a drug. This is the state of awareness, perception and being toward which I work. Its value lies in that I feel I am simultaneously both perceiving reality and being a vital part of that reality. This feeling of **wholeness** is both exceptional and gratifying. For me, it is **the** peak experience. It is the realization of two simultaneous states of being: experiencer-participant in my present incarnation, while also being the observer-witness to myself playing that role.

My main complaint—when it came my turn—was that Tammy had been cutting off and/or running away instead of attempting to communicate openly during the past weeks. As I spoke to my stashes Carole and I began to eyeball[33]. She turned into Abe Lincoln before my eyes. The resemblance between the two was fantastic. Carole, wearing black clothing, changed to the extent that not only her face but her clothing changed into Lincoln's, complete except for the missing stovepipe hat. When I reported this to Carole she connected saying that Lincoln freed the slaves as we all were doing, with her assistance, for our psyches. I felt a connection here with John Kennedy, also assassinated (the week before).

Further into the session I again encountered Carole, describing to her some spontaneous childhood experiences. She labeled them *hypnogogic imagery**, a name new to me. It is not uncommon for a very young child to feel, on the way to falling asleep, as if his or her bed were rocking. The gravitational equilibrium does something strange, as though the inner ear vestibular mechanism were not fully developed. When I, as child, was put down for a nap, in full afternoon daylight, I would lie in bed and fixate my vision on the featureless ceiling. With no visual target to focus upon, my eyes would lose their "fix" of depth perception on physical reality. My body would become dizzy and disoriented in space. Size changed. My body

---

[33] *Eyeballing* is described by W. V. Caldwell in *LSD Psychotherapy*, Grove Press, page 46:
One technique for uncovering problems. . . therapist and patient stare fixedly at one another to arouse in the patient an awareness of a variety of problems of interrelation which might not otherwise come to conscious attention.

would feel like it was shrinking at a nauseating rate. With no distinct feature to focus upon, the ceiling became something I approached at dizzying speed and as I approached its surface I could see subtle features in its surface texture. It was like orange peel or even finer like the shell texture of a hen's egg.

I speculated that maybe there was something wrong with my brain as I went through this disorienting experience time after time. Some of my playmates told me they, too, felt their beds rocking prior to sleep, so I didn't fret too much about it. I didn't talk about it with anybody and would have had a very difficult time trying to describe this experience to another. I didn't like this. I attempted, with eventual success, to control its onset. How I managed this I can't describe, except that it reminds me of biofeedback where the **tissue** itself learns a message. Either I was able to stop having these maelstrom episodes or the neurological development of my body simply outgrew them.

As I described this to Carole she encouraged me to go into such a state of consciousness. This took me unexpectedly because I had only wanted to tell her about it. So she took me through this once but my understanding of what this was and where it came from remained, at the time, void.

In researching material for this book I found a description which reverberated with my pre-nap states of consciousness. It comes from these excerpts from:
The Hidden Story of Scientology
by Omar Garrison, The Citadel Press, Secaucus, N.J:

Page 29:
   A primary goal of Dianetics is to restore the individual to full, present-time self-determination. This is accomplished by directing him back along his personal time track to contact and re-live the moments of emotion, pain, and unconsciousness that, as real or fancied threats to survival, were filed in the "red-tab" memory bank of the reactive mind.

Page 30:

   The search for the very first incident on the time track led to the discovery of prenatal engrams. Hubbard reported that the earliest could occur shortly **before conception,** and that engramic events **during** the prenatal epoch were common.

   Such a postulate meant, of course, that engrams were recorded on the cellular level. It was a highly revolutionary concept. As Hubbard himself declared, "No statement as drastic as this—as far beyond previous experience as this—can be accepted readily."

Indeed, it was not readily accepted by the scientific community at the time. However, medical researchers have since published results of their own studies which validate Hubbard's work. Upon reading this and comparing it with my youthful hypnogogic trips I underwent a classical "aha" experience. If there can be what we call "consciousness" in a single cell, which Hubbard's data supports, then why not self-consciousness within a single cell, sperm or egg? Such speculation here threatens **my** credibility. No matter to me; I have nothing to prove and no ax to grind. I have only my subjective experience to speculate on and share with you.

This scenario from Scientology so closely fits my childhood episodes that I no longer feel any puzzlement about the origin of my childhood experiences.

So what fits for me, here, is that if I put my emerging consciousness, in fantasy, into the sperm cell as it approaches and reaches the egg, I undergo exactly the same experience I had as a child. I find my body shrinking rapidly **relative to the size of the approaching egg.** I find that, upon near approach, the surface texture of the egg itself becomes visible. In the end, just before touchdown, the vastness of the egg **looms up** and swells to occupy my whole visual consciousness. As contact is made the sensation of swinging and rocking grows until my consciousness is totally lost, gone into the sea of the egg which has swallowed me. The genes fuse and never again is the sperm conscious as it once was. There is a new being to be conscious now in place of the two separate ones that existed a moment before. The sperm has undergone its death, its fulfillment, its destiny, its fusion, its metamorphosis.

Carl Jung, in his autobiography[34], writes about experiences he had at the age of seven:

I had anxiety dreams of things that were now small, now large. For instance, I saw a tiny ball at a great distance; gradually it approached, growing steadily into a monstrous and suffocating object."

In the case of this particular memory I did not obtain a sense of completion about the therapy session until years after I left formal therapy.

Our opportunities for growth and self-understanding never cease.

---

[34] Jung, Carl, *Memories, Dreams, Reflections*, 1961, page 18.

The Mad Tea Party
Tribe LSD Session of 2-29-64

Carole's many career activities kept her both busy and challenged. Between clinical activities she sandwiched the writing of professional papers, traveled to world conferences to deliver some of them, and usually had a book gestating. Her clinical activities were of at least four kinds:

First were what Carole called "talk sessions," the traditional one-on-one "50-minute hours."

Second were the one-on-one all-day LSD sessions.

Third were the weekly Tribe therapy meetings held on weekday evenings. These were four-hour round-the-circle talk sessions at which people shared their accomplishments, their screw-ups, and how they had fared, emotionally, the previous week. Some, many, of the screw-ups shocked our collective image of the person speaking. They were seen as departures from commitment to the path of growth and so we placed a heavy value judgement on such confessions. A kind of inquisition resulted. Carole, especially, and all of us in general, poked and prodded. We sought understanding and accountability; this was the serious business of ferreting out our resistances to growth and achievement. The impetus for this orientation came from Carole herself.

Fourth were the inner-Tribe all-weekend drug sessions. They were special. Typically, they were held about every six weeks.[35]

While living in Cambridge, Tammy and I could, with difficulty, partake in all but the third of these therapeutic modalities used by Carole. More than anything else, doing so meant **travel** for us. We lived almost a full day's drive or half a day's train ride (including shuttles at each end) from these exciting people.

We, but especially I, were thriving on the changes induced in us by Carole's influence on our lives. We, and especially I, got greedy for more so we elected to relocate to Bridgeport, thereby strengthening our dedication to emotional, psychological and spiritual growth. While other professionals focused upon building a career, Tammy and I chased Wholeness. This major milestone in our Tribe involvement came with our decision to relocate to Bridgeport in order to live close to Carole and Tribe.

Now, at the time of writing this book, I question the judgement of that move. While there is no doubt that we both underwent incredible self-scrutiny of behavior in relationship, this move also uprooted us from all our contacts and activities in the Cambridge area. These included Tammy's parents and my very promising career track at the Cambridge High Energy Lab. However, the

---

[35] During most of my time in therapy with Carole she had *two* ongoing Tribes, each of which met weekly for therapy. Only one of these partook in the Tribe drug sessions. Members of this inner Tribe were admonished not to leak any information about such forthcoming sessions to anyone else, especially any member of Carole's other therapy Tribe. This was to avoid exposing her to flak from an outer Tribe member who might be in "negative transference." LSD always seemed to be a source of conflict in the professional psychological community and we went to great lengths to maintain a low profile regarding our use of it.

self-scrutiny was exactly what we needed in order to learn how it was that our relationship had become such a mine field. There is no way that you can hang on to a cherished illusion when fifteen or twenty others are each giving you **their** version of reality. The blind spots of two people may overlap sometimes but the blind spots of fifteen or twenty people never will. This scrutiny was just what Tammy and I needed, so we left careers and friends to try to heal our marriage.

As I prepared to terminate one job and assume another—and as I packed our household goods—Tammy drove the car (containing our two cats and dog) down south to find us a new home. I spent a couple weeks of evenings alone in the empty house accomplishing these tasks. Finally, ready to travel south myself, I used my motorcycle to transport both it and my body to my new, and yet unseen, home. The journey had an overnight stop in Albany where I spent the night with Willard. I hadn't known him very long but Tammy and I had come to like him a lot for his warmth and sense of humor. Willard was an Israeli college student and former heroin addict.

As it happened, a Tribe LSD session was to take place the following day at Carole's home, two more hours travel for me. Willard and I left at dawn the next morning to make the last lap into Stamford and get to the session on time. So, temporarily homeless, I rode into Stamford, parked my motorcycle after a 300 mile journey, and walked into a Tribe LSD session.

Report of Session
Similar to several other Tribe sessions, this one seemed to begin several days prior to the actual scheduled beginning.

Life had been very unusual; all routines were gone and everything around me was different as I entered this session weekend. Fortunately for my emotional state I had been extremely busy doing last-minute jobs, getting furniture moved, cleaning the rented house, and finishing reports at the University laboratory.

Departing from Cambridge at early morning I was well bundled up but the first few hours were painfully cold. The ride had me full of anxiety about whether the machine would break down. Twice I skirted the edge of a dreaded rain cloud but felt only a few drops. As it got darker and colder I felt more and more depressed. Then, at midday there were two hours of warm air and sunshine. My mood swung into rapturous joy. I was certainly **feeling** all there was to be felt on that ride.

With difficulty I found Willard's place and warmed up with hot coffee. We had dinner and early to bed. Not wanting to be late for the Tribe session, we two motorcyclists left early. It was to take place at Carole's house, still two hours distant. Such conservative behavior made us the first ones to arrive.

Four women were present: Carole, Jane, Freda, and Debbie, none of whom, it was decided, took any booster. Later in the day Tammy (whom I had not seen for two weeks) came in. Being pregnant, she, of course, took none. The men all had high doses of booster except for Vic and me. Dr. George provided medical coverage. For that reason, and because he was not one of Carole's patients, he took no booster.

Ollie didn't have any but then he didn't really attend. We first had to deal with Ollie and see what was to be done with respect to him. His writing hangup surfaced again. He had not finished writing his report from our previous session and was generally in a bad way. He spoke of pulling out of the Tribe since he lived so far away and since he felt such tearing changes take place during his

transitions from session context to home-life and back.[36]
It was established that he go upstairs and write his report
until finished, with the stipulation that he was to call Carole
if he needed help. Only in that way could Carole manage
the session. Ollie accepted responsibility to communicate
any need for help and disappeared upstairs. Several hours
later he came back downstairs. His report was finished and
he looked much better.

At the stash-dump period I expressed my feeling of being
lost in time and space. Carole suggested I, therefore, take
no booster. She later surmised that it seemed there was
some residue of baggage between Ollie and me.[37] She
suggested I sever all psychic connections with Ollie then
take my half of the severed connections and roll them back
into myself. So I closed my eyes, centered myself,
conjured up the mental images and used them to get the job
done. With difficulty I finally got all the severed
connections pulled in. One big unfinished thing connecting
us was a strobe light we had built together to sell. I had to
take this machine, in fantasy, and run it through a bandsaw
so we each could have our half of it. Eat your heart out,
King Solomon!

By the time our stashes were all dumped (which seemed to
take hours) I was beginning to get a fix on space and time
and felt better. I took as much booster as I dared,

---

[36] Ollie lived near Cambridge and he had often traveled to Tribe sessions
with Tammy and me, either driving or by rail. Now that Tammy and I had moved
away from him he no longer had this support from us. Also, Ollie was the only
person in Tribe whose spouse was not also in Tribe.

[37] Ollie and I had a lot of common interests and were involved in some joint
business engineering ventures.

considering my circumstances, which was 50 micrograms (of freeform LSD).

In the Beginning there were Adam and Eve but in the beginning of this session there were Freda and I, lying on the couch in each other's arms. Then, and at this writing, I have trouble telling which couple is which. As I felt the booster take hold, our bodies seemed to melt together. As I felt the relationship become deeper and deeper I felt the strange intensity of meeting another soul completely outside the barriers of space and time. (Oh, yes, Carole had oriented this session toward JOY, and so it was.) This connection I felt with Freda seemed to take place not only in the present but also far, far back in time and far, far forward into the future. These immensely distant past and future points seemed to be one and the same. Time had become a gigantic circle, whose most distant part was where distant past met, fused with, and became distant future. This circle appeared to have a small missing segment. It was as though the recent past—Christian era, Middle Ages—had been completely 'jumped over.' These eras in time seemed filled with people who desired to meet and relate as we were doing but could not get past the barriers of cultural neurotic crud which seemed to fill their world.

At first, and very briefly, as Freda and I held each other, I got hooked on our bodies. I struggled between two conflicting ideas:
    1) Since we have bodies we should go ahead and use them, and,
    2) Sexual acting out is still a very entangling activity for people everywhere and we were not there to get ourselves entangled but just the opposite. Letting go of the sexual desire I said to myself, "Oh, well, in another lifetime, or perhaps later on in this one, but not now." As I let go of sexual desire something else opened up. I made some leap

into the meeting with Freda and it seemed that we both sailed past our bodies going far off into the cosmos together. It seemed that we had each stepped out of the ties of our present lives and had met on a level which was extra-karma[*] or above the particular plane of existence of our now-lives.

By the time Freda and I returned to earth I was so deep into the unconscious that I find it hard to describe events. I remember feeling fragmented at times, but it felt to me that it was not me who was fragmented but the rest of the world. Of course this was my projection but it didn't feel that way to me at the time.

Quentin, a brilliant mathematician and sculptor, came into Tribe because he wanted the drug experiences as much as psychotherapy. I told Quentin, "I think the whole world is going to explode!" He looked me sternly in the eye and said, "No, Trevor, I think it is **you** who are about to explode." Our eyes locked together for a long time. I had been looking for reality and/or grounding and—strange as it seems—the only place that seemed real and not delusional to me was meeting another person through our eyes. The eye contact grounded me, which is what I needed. There seemed no other reality, only visual relationship. Thanks Quentin, for that.

Next I remember lying on the grass in Carole's back yard with Quentin. We lay on our backs holding hands. My body, in contact with the soil, felt well grounded. Quentin said, "I feel as though I am on an operating table." I replied, "Yes, I feel that my right foot is being cut off." This was brief but from where in time and space did it come?

Later, still in the back yard, I sat holding hands in a circle with five others. We all were talking and, as I had felt earlier that day, I again felt the presence of the upsetting forces of the collective unconscious. I couldn't sort out how much of that came from my paranoia and how much was for real. Like eerie, unexpected gusts of wind it sometimes felt, leaving the air crackling with electricity. Feeling this during our circle, I intuitively knew that as long as we didn't break the circle and release hands in its presence nothing could happen to us.

In this circle we formed there emerged one of the most extra ordinary things I have ever experienced. The scene reminded me of **The Mad Tea Party** but at first I didn't know why. There were six people and six personalities; all of the latter were interchangeable and moved from one person to another. Our **bodies** didn't get up and move around the table to the next chair. Our personality-shell got up and moved over to the next body instead! One person had humor, another had paranoid delusions, another had joyous contact with the cosmic, another had psychic infection*, etc. None of these was strongly tied to the person it currently occupied. I assumed each of these personality-shells several times, one after the other, as they rotated around the circle.

We each must have been so psychically fluid and free that none of these personality-shells could get stuck with any individual. Also, regardless of which personality inhabited me, I could look around and clearly identify which shell anyone was 'wearing' at the moment.

The setting was Carole's back yard with its many flowers and tall ornamental grass blowing in the breeze. The whole scene resembled, and became for me, a tropical island in the Pacific. While this locale stayed fixed for me, its place in historical time did not. It wasn't enough that I "hallucinate" on peoples faces and bodies; the surroundings had to change to match the personality.

If I was watching someone who wore a 'positive'
personality their background was a tropical paradise.
Looking over at someone else who wore a negative
personality the background scene would appear to be the
same Pacific island during the time of World War II. It
would take on all the hell of war. Kurt appeared to be a
marine waiting for a Japanese bayonet to stab him in the
back. As I looked at him I felt he displayed a wariness
about acceptance of the world. Then, in the next instant, as
he looked extremely serious, Ury would say something
funny. That would break Kurt up into gales of laughter as
his serious personality was displaced by the humorous one.
Ury, a classical pianist with a wacky sense of humor, kept
the laughter moving along.

The personalities rotated around the circle faster and faster
until they (we?) became a whirlpool. This image changed
until we became a flying saucer. Again it became
important, I felt, that we keep holding hands; if anyone let
go we would all fly off into space from the centrifugal
force! It had all become an out-of-this-world scene to me.

Kurt pointed out Tammy to me; she had just arrived. I
called her over and she looked bloated and rigid to me but
as she came into the circle and became part of the nutty
goings on, she softened up. After the session we had a
warm reunion.

As a whole, this session was different. It broke up into
smaller groups of us seeking out the joy, each in our own
way, as directed. Not one time was it necessary for us to
gather and focus as a Tribe. We had no "fires to put out."
We had never achieved this at past sessions.

— end of session report —

This is how I deepened my involvement with the Tribe. . .
and what I left behind in pursuit of this involvement that
held such promise for Tammy and me.

Past Life Images

The Unexpected and the incredible belong in this world.
Only then is life whole.

— Carl Jung, *Memories, Dreams, Reflections*

The most mind-boggling thing I learned in Tribe—with the aid of LSD—is described in the following account of a transition from personal hallucination to shared experience and the implications of this transition:

During Tribe sessions there were frequent episodes of what we came to call "eyeballing." We modified Caldwell's technique, earlier described in footnote number thirty-three. Orchestrated by Carole, two Tribe members, patients **or** therapist, sat facing each other. They established and maintained constant eye contact for as long as thirty minutes. Often each would place hands on the other's shoulders while doing so. Frequently, but not always, one person was to discharge verbal hostility toward the other with growls or a stream of invectives. The remainder of the Tribe would surround this couple and watch and, under Carole's direction, "push" (psychically).

In our culture, eye contact is not held between people for long durations. It makes people uncomfortable and they break away from it before many seconds have elapsed. Not so during Carole's therapy and Tribe sessions. I learned from experience that protracted eye contact—"eyeballing" —will produce unexpected and unexplainable results often commencing in as little as thirty seconds. The face looked at undergoes changes. It is almost as if the face were made of modeling clay and an invisible sculptor were rapidly reshaping it. The form of the face could become virtually anything face-like. I have seen faces change into images of people from other cultures and other times, into images from mythology and folklore. It could become a wizened, ancient Chinese man, an atavistic savage, an Eskimo, a werewolf, an animal, a Nordic woman, a Biblical character or a black African. The face might look like a Picasso painting with part of it in profile and part frontal view—a fascinating image. Sometimes the face changes rapidly from one image to another; sometimes one image appears and stays fixed.

When I first observed this phenomenon, in my early LSD therapy sessions before entering Carole's Tribe, and later during my early Tribe sessions, I had assumed that they were simply my drug-induced hallucinations. I had already watched my image, reflected in a hand mirror, undergo incredible (and often repulsive) changes under LSD. Also, photographs of my family members, in this therapy, were not even static. During my early Tribe sessions I learned that these facial changes were not restricted to the couple who were eyeballing. When I was one of those surrounding the couple, watching the face of one of them, I would also see the face appear to change. This was still another manifestation of LSD hallucinations, or so I thought at the time.[38]

As I said earlier, Tribe members were required to submit a written report on each session attended. In addition, Carole imposed another requirement on us: before anyone could

---

[38] John Lilly, on page 88 of *John Lilly, So Far*, offers:

"John drew the conclusion that the term hallucination is rather meaningless, a trash heap for a wide variety of potentially significant experiences that are not acceptable according to established systems of belief. In the light of this line of reasoning, psychiatry begins to appear startlingly unscientific."

attend a drug session she or he must have read everyone else's report on the previous session. This communication structure was absolute.

During Tribe sessions there is more going on than is verbalized. People have feelings, thoughts, intuitions, and sensations that frequently don't get reported at the moment because to do so would be to interrupt something. These things frequently found their way into the written reports that were created a few days following. When the reports were subsequently read by the rest of Tribe attention was called to these unspoken feelings, intuitions and perceptions for the first time by their authors. Imagine my astonishment when I read others' reports that described perceptions of faces changing into the **very same** images that I perceived at the time! When I observed, for example, Quentin's face change into that of an aged Oriental woman, I might have read later that several others saw the identical image appear on Quentin's face during the same event. My personal hallucination was no longer just mine! Could there be such a thing as a shared hallucination? If so, what was it and how does one explain it? I puzzled over this enigma for several months. One evening, during a Saturday Tribe party at Frank and Freda's house, I mentioned this puzzlement to Frank. He responded by walking to his bookshelf and handing me a booklet by Edgar Cayce[39]. In it I read a description of a friend of his who could see auras:

If I am talking to a person and he makes a statement of opinion which reflects a prejudice gained in one of his former lives, I see as he speaks a figure in his aura, which is a reflection of the personality he was in that time—I see, that is, the figure of a Greek, or an Egyptian, or whatever he

---

[39] Cayse, Edgar, *Auras; An Essay On The Meaning Of Colors*, A.R.E. Press, Virginia Beach, VA

happened to be. As soon as we pass on to another subject and the opinion gained in that incarnation passes, the figure disappears. Later he will express another view. Perhaps he will say, "I have always loved Italy and wanted to go there," and as he speaks I will see the figure of a Renaissance man or an old Roman. During the course of an afternoon's conversation I may see six or eight of these figures.

Frank is an electrical engineer who designs microwave antennas. He is conservative in taste and interests so I was surprised that his library would extend to something this far afield from his turf.

This was my first exposure to the ideas of Cayce. It lead me to the library where I found more writings about the man and his life. I found another description that was similar to my own:

The unconscious mind, the readings of Cayce explained, retains the memory of every experience through which the individual has passed—not only from the time of birth, but also before birth in all its previous experiences. These pre-birth memories exist below what might be called a trap door, and at deeper levels of the unconscious mind than those commonly tapped by modern psychotherapists.[40]

Either Carole's dynamics or the effect of LSD was capable of reaching deeper levels of the unconscious mind ". . . than those commonly tapped by modern psychotherapists."

The concept and description of Cayce's past life readings was vivid. Discussed were ideas of past lives and reincarnation, and in his work I found a model of reality that explained, exactly, my dilemma of our "shared hallucinations."

I was instantly converted into a believer of the model of past lives, reincarnation and karma—not as an act of

---

[40] Cerminara, Gina, *Many Lives, Many Loves*, page 64, Wm Sloan Assoc.

faith—but from my own experience under LSD.[41]
According to the Cayce model, then, the face changes we
"saw" were residual images of the individual's past lives.

As Cayce's aura-reading friend implied and as I discovered,
a drug is not necessary to induce this experience. Now I
see faces change with anyone with whom I maintain protracted eye contact. When I do this with people who are
casual acquaintances I have found a strong correlation here:
When the person holds eye contact long enough for me to
begin to see a change in his face, that is the precise instant
when he breaks eye contact with me. I now believe that
this strange perception is spontaneous and happens to both
people simultaneously. When it begins it usually arouses
fear in people. They break off eye contact out of their
discomfort at seeing what is "not supposed to be there."
This is something that people rarely allow and almost never
discuss. (After all, we have been carefully taught, "It is
impolite to stare.") Probably the fear is simply fear of the
unknown or fear of losing control or going insane. Perhaps
they intuitively know that they are revealing a part of
themselves that they are a stranger to, that is, that resides in
their unconscious mind only. Then to disclose it to another
is to bestow some manner of power to the other. In reality
there is nothing at all to fear from watching another's face
change. It is a deeper level of human contact on the
psychic level. I find it fascinating to share the experience
with a close friend and we each learn something when we
allow it to happen. To me it is both a path to self-enlight-
enment and to developing a stronger bond with a friend or
loved one. The more integrated the personality and the

---

[41] Lilly, John, op. cit., page 175:

"Many of those who turned to spiritual experiences after using LSD in the 1960's
and 1970's turned to esoteric traditions to provide a context from which they could
gain a better perspective on what had happened to them."

more experience one has with inner growth, the easier it seems to be to allow the eyeballing experience.

Food for thought is provided by Julian Jaynes[42] as he speculates on the significance of eye-idols. These were found by the thousands on a branch of the Euphrates river and have thin cracker-like bodies surmounted by eyes, dating from 3,300 B.C. They were carved in alabaster and once tinted with malachite paint. Like the earlier Gerzean and Amatrian tusk idols of Egypt, they may be held in the hand.

He theorizes from these the extreme importance of eye-to-eye contact:

The development of such eye-to-eye contact into authority relationships and love relationships is an exceedingly important trajectory that has yet to be traced.

. . . you are more likely to feel a superior's authority when you and he are staring straight into each other's eyes. There is a kind of stress, an unresolvedness about the experience, and within something of a diminution of consciousness, so that, were such a relationship mimicked in a statue, it would enhance the hallucination of divine speech.

Here Jaynes describes the voice of God speaking through the eyes of what the statues represent. The theme of his book, in fact, is that, prior to the development of what we call **consciousness,** God communicated to people by speaking to them through some inner voice. This was often triggered by eye contact.

These "idols that speak" are found in many ancient cultural artifacts including excavations in Turkey, the upper and middle branches of the Euphrates, and early Mesopotamia.

---

[42] See Jaynes, *The Origin of Consciousness in the Breakdown of the Bicameral Mind* pages 168-171, Houghton Mifflin Co.

Catskill Spook Session
Tribe Mescaline* of 10-31-64

Tammy and I flew to the north country early. I had some work to do at the Cambridge High Energy Physics Lab. and spent two days there. Once in Boston, we had lunch at our favorite tea house. Afterward, window shopping, I saw a gauze and wire butterfly which I bought on impulse.

Everyone assembled at Dr. Larry and Lisa's place, way up in Catskill County, on time. They had a rural home with lots of open space and no neighbors; noise would not be an issue. Larry, a psychiatrist, provided the necessary medical coverage for our drug use.

Tammy and I had not met sexually for several days. Friday evening we met twice in a thirty minute period. I remarked to Tammy that we had violated one of the cardinal rules of the psychedelic experience as voiced by several "authorities"—namely, to "avoid sexual congress prior to the trip for an enlightening experience." I didn't believe this and it turned out to be, for both Tammy and me, not so. The way I see it is that sexual congress is so guilt provoking for most people that its avoidance serves to keep the person guilt-free from this source. It is not sexual congress that should be avoided but the acquisition of guilt!

Dr. Larry brought some magic mushrooms: Amanita Muscaria!

Friday night stash-dump went well except for Kurt, who made noises about never again obeying the irrational—and he bugged everybody with it.

Saturday morning stash-dump was prolonged. We had ample time so no matter. Kurt spoke of the session's themes: **All Saints' Day** and **divorce.** He read a spine chilling account of Holy Evening, the precursor to Halloween. Then he read the dictionary's definition of divorce. In our discussion the subject shifted to *work* and what it is. Paula, our aspiring opera singer, had trouble with the concept. I suggested someone read from *The Prophet,* the passage on *work*, which Carole did. During the reading I watched Paula. She seemed quite moved by it and it seemed to speak to her on an unfamiliar level, especially when she heard, "Work is love made visable."

Jane led stash-dump, Tammy said a prayer, and Dr. Larry passed out the pieces of mushroom. They were too small to have much effect except on a symbolic level. Dr. Larry spoke of the history and meaning of the fungus. To me it felt and tasted somewhat like raw abalone. Neither pleasant nor unpleasant, the mushroom was different from anything I had ever eaten.

Carole then passed out the main booster, mescaline. I had three hundred milligrams plus ten milligrams of methedrine. I felt the drugs beginning to work in thirty minutes. This is about the same time as the onset of the LSD experience. I felt comfortable until I heard Ury heaving in the kitchen. After that I felt slightly nauseous with body reaction to the alkaloid chemicals. In a few minutes this passed.

Awaiting the onset of the drug experience, we lay in a large circle. Carole was in the center and all our feet touched her body while she read more from *The Prophet* by Gibran. This is a special book and it always moves me emotionally (all of us in Tribe, really) to hear a portion of it.

Ingrid, a gorgeous lady attorney on whom I had developed a crush, had a beautiful, black, unembellished, floppy hat and we created some fun with it. One by one, it sat on all our heads. With each person we projected onto the face/hat combination. It made a wonderful frame for each face as our perception became altered with the drug. It was a sharing of projections—of hallucinations. As others projected images I could quickly feel a grasp of and understand the perceiver's position. Following that understanding I was in a position to embellish the image and it would be picked up by the others.

At the time, Tammy was breast-feeding four-month-old Thea, the daughter we would never have had save for Carole keeping our marriage intact this long. Carole suggested that we in Tribe sample Tammy's breast milk. Tammy was shy about exposing her "floppy tits" but we were universal in disallowing her to avoid fulfilling her Tribe "mother" role. Of course, Kurt was first in line. Ingrid, sitting next to me, offered, "I would like to try that but I haven't the courage." My response was to place her second in line after Kurt. She drank milk and returned absolutely glowing. We related for a time and I discovered how much Ingrid turns me on at all levels: physically, psychically, sexually, intellectually, the works. Ingrid said she wanted more milk. I said, "Let's go get some." By then, Dr. Larry was on top of Tammy and Ingrid didn't want to disturb them. I said, "Nonsense, if you need nourishment from Mamma you have to go and make your needs known and horn in if necessary. This is a Tribe thing, not something exclusively for Mamma and Papa." As we walked over to them I told Ingrid she was acting like she was walking in on her parents in the middle of a screw—to which she agreed. She grabbed one of Tammy's breasts and I grabbed the other. Dr. Larry and Tammy were not only cooperative but delighted as well, as we took nourishment from Mamma Tammy.

Later Dr. Larry asked me, "Can you help Lisa?" Larry's
wife, Lisa, was a nurse. I have a thing for nurses; I
married one once, remember? I went over to her and lay
down beside her. I asked her if she was OK and she said
she was but she seemed glad to be near someone. I was
lying on the floor; Lisa lay on top of me. Occasionally I
sensed that she would retreat from the intimacy. I asked
her to stay with the flow. She wanted to change positions.
She wanted me on top so she couldn't "run away." By this
time my mescaline was coming on full force. After a while
I began to feel a sense of sharp hostility. I thought it
coming from Lisa but I wasn't certain. Trying to ascertain
its source and meaning, I let myself feel it for a while.
There was a lot of activity going on around the room with
people's dynamics. Did what I feel come from Lisa, me,
or some others around the room? I began to see a pattern.
As Lisa would open up I would feel a surge of sexuality
coming on in my body. It would come smoothly and
quickly and build up in intensity. Then, at a particular
point it would stop. This happened several times and I
perceived that Lisa would allow the sexual feelings to grow
either until she became conscious of them or until they
reached a threatening level, then she would stop the flow. I
didn't realize it yet but I was beginning to 'read' what was
going on in her unconscious. Imagery came to me about
what **might** have been going on in her. Tentatively I told
her about what I felt I sensed in her. It felt right to me but
I was uncertain that it was not something I was getting
from my own dynamics or from someone else in the room.
My imagery of what I felt got stronger and stronger and I
felt certain it came from Lisa. Suddenly, I intuitively
realized she had a brother. When asked about this she
affirmed the fact. What came to me was that I was
standing in for her brother—feelingwise—in some past time
incident. She and her brother had a strong mutual
attraction, about which Lisa felt guilty, as I read it. She

and her brother had shared sexual feelings (probably frequently), as we do in Tribe, with lots of bodily contact but with no penetration. All this had to be disguised as 'wrestling' whenever observed by their parents. This was, for Lisa, the root of her inability to clearly sort out sexuality and hostility.

Earlier in this book I related how Kurt had once described my repressed memory. It took place years prior to this Halloween event, at one of my LSD sessions in Carole's office. I had regressed into my childhood. During the day Carole and Kurt saw me, several times, inexplicably chewing on my lower lip. They didn't know what to make of it. Finally Kurt closed his eyes and began to describe a scene that had taken place in my childhood. I was amazed to hear Kurt describe what had happened to me. I had repressed the entire thing but as he described and unveiled the scene, word by word, I knew it to be accurate. The repressed memory flowed back to consciousness as I listened. This was one of the most astonishing things I ever experienced. Another person who had no prior knowledge of my past was telling me what resided, repressed, in my memory bank. Talk about ESP!

Now, at Catskill, for the first time in my life I was 'reading' the unconscious of another in the way Kurt earlier had read mine.

Still with Lisa, I saw another scene in my mind: There was a beach, at night, with an amusement park nearby. I mentioned this to her and she said, "I had just been thinking about the beach!" The scene I saw was Lisa and her brother and several of his friends. All the friends were having sex with Lisa and a good time was had by all . . . except that all the stimulus caused Lisa to somehow psychically explode. Her brother picked up all the pieces of her psyche and put them back together for her.

Ingrid came over and the three of us lay together. I got a new set of imagery and thought it was from Ingrid. I saw her with her father. They were engaged in some sort of "wrestling" with a strong flow of sexuality. Then her father had an orgasm. This event flipped him into a strong guilt feeling about sex with his daughter and he reacted by slapping her in order to keep himself from feeling the responsibility for his part in the sex play. I described this whole scene to Ingrid and she replied, "That's right." I told her that it wasn't her fault and that there had been no reason or basis for her punishment except in terms of her father's unconscious.

Later, again with Lisa, I picked up an intense feeling of hostility from her. It was mostly for Dr. Larry, I felt, but was also for her father from past time. I shared my imagery with her. The intensity of the emotion I was picking up, I told her, was so strong it could be dangerous and I said I was concerned for her safety if she didn't get it expressed somehow. She replied that any expression of it would get turned inward on herself. I felt this needed more insight than I had and called for Carole. Carole was busy elsewhere so Ollie came over and he verified my feelings on every point. To us, Lisa appeared to have herself in a straight-jacket of physical control. She seemed, to me, to have so much hostility that she felt any expression of it would put her so out of control that she **had** to contain it. I began to feel knives in my body and I told her that I was in pain. I said I wanted her to spit at me and get some of the hostility discharged and if she did this I would be free of this pain. She was resistant but willing to work hard and did manage to spit some. She did better at verbal expression of hostility. I tried to teach her the distinction between hostility (a feeling) and destructiveness (acts). She began to understand that the hostility didn't belong to her but to the relationship and that it must be discharged in nondestructive ways.

During her hostility discharge my perception of her began to change. She began to look like an elephant! At first I didn't know what to make of this or whether to share my perception. It persisted and I said to myself, "It must have meaning or it wouldn't be there," so I simply said to Lisa, "You look like an elephant." It seemed so out of context that I almost giggled. I noticed a trace of a smile on Lisa's face. Ollie, still trying to get her to express hostility, said to her, "He called you an elephant; how does that make you feel?" She smiled even more. I began, partly in jest, to describe what the image meant to me. I said she must have been an elephant in her last incarnation. The animal appeared to be female and was definitely an Indian elephant. I said that my feeling of India and its culture was one of male supremacy and that Lisa had chosen to be an elephant because she had misperceived the trunk for a penis. I felt that the only female in that culture to be respected was the female elephant due to the sheer bulk and strength of the beast. Ollie said that Lisa, as an elephant, had been all blown up with her "ponderousity." By this time the mood and atmosphere had shifted to humor. I ordered Lisa to become a butterfly in her next incarnation in order to once more bring the universe into harmony and balance. I cautioned her not to misperceive the worm in the cocoon to be her final form and not to try to fly until her wings had dried out in the sunshine.

At this point I recalled that I had bought, without knowing why, a gauze butterfly that morning. I went and fetched it and handed it to Lisa. She didn't know how I had known to bring it and I didn't either. Lisa now looked much better to Ollie and me.

Later, Carole, Dr. Larry and Lisa made arrangements for Lisa to come down south for a session; then I felt OK about her. She still had a lot of psychic stuff to carry but arrangements had been made for her.

At session's end there was much play and joy. Ury at the piano and Quentin at drums made wonderful music. Ingrid and I swam in the pool. Good feelings abounded. It was a day of fun and rewarding hard work for me. Wonderful, wonderful session.

Appearance of My Anima*
Dream of 11-11-64

*On a hilltop, overlooking a small village, I was with
several or most of Tribe. It was a beautiful day. We
collectively watched a strange sight: We could actually see
the air over the scene—starting from several miles away.
The air would become wind and the wind would converge
until a small whirlwind would form. This happened several
times and the wind was, somehow, an embodiment of
cosmic consciousness or, perhaps, a physical representation
of cosmic unity. Each time this happened we each felt that
fantastic feeling of cosmic unity within ourselves. With the
last of these, the whirlwind came right into our midst and
from the filmy, smoky quality of the wind there solidified
the form of a young woman. She was, I felt, an
embodiment of the cosmic—now in the solid form of flesh
and blood. She was very beautiful but rather big-boned
and not light and airy as I would have thought. Possibly
she was a Slavic-peasant type. She was dressed like
Cinderella—in a sparkling white dress—as if she stepped
out of a fairy tale.*

*There was something strange about her. Something about
her sexual feelings was repressed and had been running
her. Perhaps she had been molested when she was young
and, as a result, carried a repression? Prior to her arrival
in the midst of Tribe, we knew she would be coming and
we also knew about her autonomous complex. Tribe members took a vote as to whether to put her to the test of
confronting her complex. Except for Don, we voted to do*

94

*so. Don, alone, voted not to. So there she was, now, with
Tribe. We went inside a house and she walked into the
kitchen and I followed her there. It seemed a good opportunity to go through the thing we voted on. As she was
occupied with something I approached her from behind and
put my arms around her waist. Then I slid my hands down
toward her crotch. As soon as she felt the downward
motion of my hands she flipped out of what she had been
doing and her complex began to run her. She guided my
hands inside her dress and against her bare skin as they
slid down. During the few seconds it took for my hands to
reach her vulva she was so deep into her sexual complex
that her clit was hard and her labia already wet. I stroked
her vulva for two or three seconds and in that short
duration she came and simultaneously urinated all over,
completely out of control. During this scene Carole was in
the kitchen with us and had observed what the young
woman had gone through.*

The **anima** is described by Jung as "the feminine part of a
man's soul."[43] The woman, with whom I felt a strong
identification in this dream, comes across as my anima.
The whole scene was dripping with sexual symbolism
which I felt as both man and woman. This woman was a
part of my own psyche. Tribe voted to confront "her" with
her complex which was to bring her repression to consciousness and thereby heal her. In coming to acceptance
with the female side of my psyche I was learning to be
joyfully androgynous.

---

[43] Jung, Carl, *The Archetypes and the Collective Unconscious*, 1959, page
59, Vol 9, part 1, collected works.

Carole as Collective Tribe Unconscious

She was like one of those seers who is at the same time a strange animal, like a priestess in a bear's cave. Archaic and ruthless as truth and nature. . . what she said at these moments was so true and to the point that I trembled before it.

— Carl Jung, writing about his mother's personality,
in *Dreams, Memories, Reflections* page 50.

Carole was heavily guided by input from her highly talented intuition. I, being a visually dominated person, saw this intuition as an image of a pipeline coming down from above entering the base of her skull. When this pipeline fed her data about a patient with whom she was working, her eyes would gleam with sudden understanding. Her determination was then redoubled to steer the patient toward that part of his or her growth which was being resisted.

Carole's intuition had maximum data to back it up. Since the doorway to Tribe was open only to patients, every person in Tribe was also her patient. Each of us had spent many hours with her in the most intimate possible conversation yielding our innermost thoughts, desires, and secrets at her expert probing. She gave us LSD which opened the doorway to the unconscious. She knew things about each of us—our repressions—that we ourselves didn't know. She knew our talents, addictions, needs, desires, aversions, habits, prejudices, attitudes, and guilts. She knew our strengths and weaknesses. We freely gave her this knowledge for we each had sought her healing power. Her knowledge, of this depth and breadth, of each Tribe member gave Carole immense power over our individual and collective lives. No one else on Earth had accumulated such a store of information. With this knowledge came her power to orchestrate our lives and feelings, which she did with great vigor.

In the personality model of the late psychiatrist Carl Jung, we each have four attributes:
Thought, Feeling, Sensation and **Intuition.** Of these, the last two are functions of taking in information, while the first two are functions of sizing up that information.

Sensation and **intuition** are perceptive. Sensation is perceiving with our five senses what is in our shared world-at-large.[44] One's conscious mind has no input beyond sensation. Intuition is our private information channel from our unconscious mind and from the collective unconscious mind of our culture.

Thought and **feeling** are judgmental in nature. They serve to determine what we do about our perceptions—ultimately to either approach or avoid.

Intuitive insights come through the unconscious mind and hence are neither predictable nor reproducible. Being outside of cause and effect they are ignored or denied by classical science.

Carole has been gifted with the richness of a nonstop intuition and it is one of her greatest strengths. Intuitive inputs, unlike sensory inputs, cannot be directly shared with

---

[44] Actually, your experience of the world-at-large is your experience of the inner re-creation of it that your mind fabricated based upon the sum total of all your sensory inputs plus whatever distortions may have occurred to these impressions on their way to you.

another. They come from strictly private places in one's mind. They are indirectly shared, one to another, by verbal or written report without possibility of confirmation. They are, therefore, subject to distortion by the person reporting either from personal prejudice (unconscious distortion) or from deliberate intent to deceive (conscious distortion.) Because of this potential for distortion we learn to be skeptical of someone's announcement of a 'hunch.' We learn from experience who is accurate in reporting intuitive knowledge and who is not. We learn from experience who tends to lie and who does not. We learn because after the fact (and to our dismay) it becomes revealed when someone has, earlier, lied or otherwise offered an inaccurate evaluation.

A highly intuitive psychotherapist such as Carole can function with incredible depth and precision. She can achieve therapeutic goals unreachable by non-intuitive therapists. Such people, I suspect, are rarities. When I met Carole I was twenty-seven years old and I had never met anyone remotely like her before. She could read me like an open book and she could comprehend how my mind worked. Until then I had been a puzzle to my parents, teachers and others. Here, at last, I had found a teacher competent to guide me through the labyrinth of my very active and volatile unconscious mind. Early in my relationship with Carole, when we discussed something or other, she said, "You have some reservation, what is it?" To my astonishment I realized that she was correct, and also that I hadn't myself even been in touch with the fact that I had a reservation! In hindsight this seems unremarkable, but at the time I was highly gratified to find someone who could tell me what I was thinking even when I couldn't myself do so. So I learned to open up to and trust Carole's intuitions. I trusted her freedom from prejudice and I trusted her integrity not to distort her readings from intent to deceive.

As I learned to trust Carole's intuitive authority in guiding me through my personal psychotherapy so did the others in her Tribe. By knowing each of us so intimately, she could play us, one against another, in mix-and-match relationships. She would assign one to spend time with whomever she thought could best catalyze his or her growth. These assigned relationships could be centered around anything imaginable: a work project, sharing children, living together, having a sexual relationship, a student/teacher set-up, or a periodic check-in special authority to help another stay on a difficult track in life. As her Tribe grew in size, Carole acquired a large stockpile of personality types from which to draw. For example, suppose a patient's current psycho-dynamics centered on repressed feelings from a neurotic childhood relationship with a fearsome uncle. Carole would ask, "Who among us looks most to you like your uncle?" The person named would then be brought into some encounter or relationship with the patient. This was done to provoke—in the service of the patient's therapy—much as rubbing a match across its striking surface provokes a rapid expansion of flame.

What might happen if the integrity of the therapist is ruptured and this power gets misused? What happens when your highly intuitive therapist allows a breach in her integrity? Information from her totally private intuitive pipeline starts coming out distorted, that is what happens. How are people who have long trusted in her intact integrity to learn of this new situation? I can only answer for myself and from years of hindsight. The learning, of course, arises out of comparing the outcomes with the predictions. The problem with learning by this means is that it is a long, slow process; it takes years. Carole began to make predictions about me which no longer coincided with the months-later ultimate outcomes. For example, before Thea was born I asked Carole if she thought it would be a boy or a girl. Carole replied, "Oh, it will be a boy, no doubt about it." She even put this in writing in a letter she later sent to me. Now, there is nothing wrong with making an incorrect prediction but to qualify the prediction with "no doubt about it" leaves one to wonder when it turns out to be incorrect.

Additionally, she began to lose credibility when she stated her occasional incorrect opinion as though it were a fact not to be argued with. For example, we were selecting pen names for ourselves for a Tribe book. Each person was to write one chapter. Carole chose "Destiny" for her pen name. I said that I wanted mine to be "Arjuna." Carole said in a huff, "You can't use that; **it isn't even a name.**" If I had felt like making an issue of it—which I didn't—I could have told her that "Arjuna" is the name of the leading figure in the Bhagavad Gita. This Indian scripture is three thousand years old, give or take a century, and so is the name.

It started slowly. In fact, the first few times I noticed that she had missed her mark, there was no **pattern** there for me to see. Over the years, however, I began to watch her track record with me and with others. I watched her performance progressively deteriorate. As I see it, she filled this performance void, vigorously and aggressively, with demands that we not question her innate "authority."

In doing this she began to replace her pronouncements of therapeutic brilliance with statements that didn't seem to ring as true as they had in the past. With twenty-twenty hindsight, I see the deterioration of my marriage running parallel in time with the deterioration in Carole's helpfulness to me. This is not to say that Carole contributed to the demise of my marriage; on the contrary she heroically worked to keep it going for five years. It does mean that her value to me as a life-guide began to run down.

Once I was discussing this with Dr. Larry and he mentioned a time he saw as critical in her redirecting her path. This took place in Carole's living room on a Saturday carbogen[45] session. As Dr. Larry described the scene it came into clear recall for me, too. I had watched the events Dr. Larry described but unlike him, in my naivety, I did not see the significance of them.

There were two medical doctors present, Larry and George. The living room floor was strewn with supine people and the carbogen gas bottle was being passed around. Carole and one or both doctors managed the passing. I watched Carole, supine on the carpet, place the carbogen mask on her face. She shortly took it off and reported to all present that she encountered nothing but "junk." A few minutes later she, once again, went under the carbogen; once again, she came back and reported there was nothing there for her but "the same junk: images only of playing cards". She refused a third confrontation with her unconscious material. Having no way to understand this, I simply concluded that there was a reasonable explanation, somewhere, for Carole's unwillingness to return to the bottle of carbogen to meet a need for completion. It is now my conviction that, within the framework of psychological growth in which Carole lived, there was no such explanation. Simply put, as I see it, she copped out to her fear. She didn't do what she had all the rest of us doing with our personal fear: confronting it; instead she withdrew.

---

[45] Carbogen and its effects are fully described in a following chapter.

Looking back at this part of my life, this was the greatest tragedy. My feeling is one of grief that Carole, for want of courage, did not attain what I saw as her potential for becoming a leading-edge healer of the personality.

Purity of Heart is to Will One Thing
Tribe LSD Session; 3-13-65

A *ceremony* is a series of acts, often symbolically prescribed by law, custom or authority, in matters of religion or state. A *ritual* is a form of conducting worship.

These things were, I had believed, static and unchanging. This belief I felt to have derived from my early religious training. My dictionary only implies that they are unchanging by describing them as "historical." We hear ritual being read from centuries-old books. Ritual serves as a bridge into experiences not usually felt. It reminds us of the aliveness of our spiritual world which we forget in our daily mundane lives of boiled potatoes and parking meters.

This—mostly unconscious—spirit world is part of every culture, yet each culture's rituals differ from those of its neighbor. It is the details of the ritual which differ while the feelings aroused by the ritual are, I think, similar for all. Every culture creates its own ritual path to the spirit. My father was an atheist and he had his ritual of denial. His mother, my grandmother, was heavily into the Methodist Church and it was to these contradictory rituals I was exposed. While my father became an atheist out of rebellion against his mother, I had an opportunity to observe the extremes they embodied. This was one of the many conflicts I brought to therapy, and I was left with the belief that ritual was changeless and encrusted. Carole's Tribe ritual, in contrast to this, is ever in a state of flux. Creative ideas are woven into the scenario of a session's ritual. Some are effective and become used again; others are passed over. We don't need ritual as a bridge to the unconscious because our orientation, dedication and boosters melt the wall between conscious and unconscious. We use ritual—created or borrowed—for its sheer beauty and inspiration. The colors, the smells, the touches, the sounds—all the sensations aroused by our ritual—stimulate our neural passages and open our psyches. Each session has its ritual authorities chosen before the event. These people gather, brainstorm, and create a scenario for the session's ritual.[46]

The Friday night preceding the session the Tribe met at the local jazz night club where Patrick and his jazz trio were playing. His music seemed exceptionally beautiful. From there we drove up the mountain to Lake Cloverleaf. We arrived at the borrowed lodge late at night and in deep snow. I felt vibrant and alive and, until 3:00 AM, I felt wide awake and was ready to start the session then and there. As we had more people than beds I finally bedded down with Ollie. Tammy arrived early in the morning with infant Thea and they climbed in next to us.

The session didn't begin until about noon but we had all weekend so lateness wasn't an issue. The theme, **Purity of Heart is to Will One Thing,** has its origin in the work of existential writer Sören Kierkegaard.

As ceremony authority, I began by instructing everyone to search outside for fifteen minutes. They were to find that which symbolized the one thing willed which would lead to purity of heart, and to bring it back to share as an

---

[46] As a 1966 Christmas gift, I received a book from Carole: *Shamanism; Archaic Techniques of Ecstasy*, by Mircea Eliade. This cloth edition of 610 pages is both scholarly and universal in coverage. She inscribed it admonishing me to learn from it new techniques of ecstacy for Tribe.

expression of feeling. I brought back a live branch and a dead branch from the same shrub. I announced that I willed **consciousness and light.** To me they represented one thing and Tribe accepted them as such. Some people didn't say what they willed. Perhaps their expression was nonverbal but I thought they avoided the direct request. Perhaps it would be their undoing but it didn't feel important. Willard returned late with his object; he later told me it was because he got lost in the snow. (After the session he got lost again driving home.)

I took fifty micrograms of LSD. Quentin directed the session and was wonderful doing so. He told a fairy tale about the sound of the human voice. His orientation toward the irrational was fantastic, beautiful and fun. My booster made it hard to stay focused on the story but this is how it is with boosters. I resisted the desire to float off into somewhere, to disconnect from the activity in the room. I knew there would be time for that later if it was in the cards. I found myself wanting to add bits and pieces to the fairy tale.

Quentin directed us to relate and just **feel.** I remember coming into contact with Ingrid. As soon as we touched I felt an updraft hit us. We held each other for a few minutes and together we soared around the cosmos bumping into assorted satellites that now clutter the universe. What was so astonishing to me was the strong and immediate result of Ingrid and me touching: the uplifting we each experienced. When I had touched other people I had no such feeling. Ingrid and I spoke with Paula about our mutual buoyancy and invited her to soar with us. She joined our hug, quickly followed by Don who made a fourth. We began to experiment with different elevations. Paula began laughing and making jokes. All three of us told her that she was resisting the mystical experience. I didn't have to surmise her resistance; I could **see** and **feel** its reality. For this reason I had no hesitation at telling her about it (as I might had I thought I might have misread her.) Paula left her resistance on the ground as we four lifted off again. Our four-way flight seemed to attract others who migrated toward our soaring pile. Soon we were about a dozen glued-together people all psychically traveling through the astral together in one huge hug. Two thoughts came to me that felt important to us here: 1), The dissolving of my identity and letting go of it, and 2), The resulting birth of a Tribe identity.

A strong visual image came to me as this pile grew in strength. A childbirth was taking place in a grand cathedral. This, to the thinking part of me, was a contradiction; children are born in hospitals or homes, not cathedrals. My spiritual side saw nothing contradictory here. This scene appeared quite natural, in fact, for the cathedral represents the soul and spirit. What better place, in personal or collective fantasy, for an old soul to newly emerge from a womb in new flesh?

In spite of my early conditioning and prejudice about the historical invalidity of organized religion, I knew that my imaginary cathedral was committed to the spiritual well-being of its people and was solid and good. I saw this child as a spiritual offspring of our Tribe.

As people migrated toward our collective fusion the vertical mass hug somehow metamorphosed into a horizontal mass human puddle. When several people are lying in a pile, bodies are draped over other bodies in several layers. If your body happens to be somewhere in the middle or bottom of the pile it becomes practically immobilized and, at the same time, feels somewhat squashed by the weight of surrounding bodies. Fingers and toes may be wiggled but nothing else. This, not unlike one of Carole's "mummifications," evokes claustrophobic fear in me; under this influence I move toward a panic state. Feeling a sharp pain in an arm or leg, or perhaps struggling hard to breathe, I would let go of it along with the desire to move. The panic would then evaporate. The letting go refers to the particular part of my body in distress. With the letting go of these several body parts came a feeling of dissociation in space. It felt as though my body parts had come unglued and were floating away from one another. I couldn't identify with these floating parts; they weren't part of me. I was unable to discriminate between my floating body parts and the bodies of the others in the pile. It was a process of letting go of my identity and flowing with Tribe feelings. The birth in the cathedral, I felt, was able to come into being because each of us on the pile had relinquished our personal identities as we surrendered to something greater.

This is difficult to describe because the concepts of **I** and **me** lost meaning both during the event and as I attempt to write about it. When I yielded my ego to the Tribe Identity there was no **I**. Yet, I was conscious of the experience and remember it vividly. I felt free to move in space and time yet instead chose to stay with the Tribe Identity. In doing this I felt carried to new times and places as part of the collective Tribe entity (through which I perceived). The most memorable of these was meeting a "man" from another planet, or perhaps this was an entity unfettered by space/time physics and who didn't even need a planet. I felt a new and highly creative relationship crystallizing. This meeting felt delicate, and clarity of perception and action struck me as critical. Any misperception between him and us felt like it could lead to mutual destruction. We are made of matter. If this other were made of anti-matter then we would explode on contact. This meeting intuitively felt significant.

We Earth creatures, who are so universally neurotic, have universal identity hangups. We identify with the ego—the core of the neurosis—and that part of us we cannot accept we project onto another. Our neurotic projective mechanism is so universal that we had to undergo a test situation in order to tell if we were clear enough to meet this entity. In this case our test might have been our willingness to forgo individual ego identity for Tribe identity.

The Vulnerability of Violence
Dream of 5-10-65

This dream had two levels. The first was a movie I
watched; later into it I was **in** the movie itself and that
interior adventure became the reality of the dream.

*First I dreamed of the Tribe. In it Carole and I discussed
how people looked to us. The only one of these I clearly
remembered was Ury. I said he looked like a grieving old
man.*

*Next I was to watch over a young woman to keep her from
fragmenting (dissociating), much as some people are to
watch over others during a session.*

*I took this woman to a movie and we sat to watch it. I felt
strongly attracted to her. I was looking forward to
smooching it up with her later on if the opportunity
presented itself.*

*I knew that the movie stared William Holden although I
never saw him on screen. The plot, strange and startling,
was about people of the Earth and their fighting each
other. There was shown a series of civil wars and small
"brush-fire" wars springing up. This is as it always was.*

*Then, at a critical moment, all the people were somehow
given a secret: if someone attacked you and you were able
to get hold of one of the attacker's spent bullets (that was
not too damaged), you could learn something from that
bullet which gave you the power to kill your attacker with
your very next shot. This was certain; there was big power*

*in the spent bullet. So when a battle started with near
misses by both sides it lasted only until one side or the
other managed to locate an intact, spent bullet from its opponent. Then it was all over, or nearly so, for the other
side. It didn't have to be a bullet; it could be any object
used by your opponent to try and kill you.*

*The spent bullet gave one the power to kill off a whole
band of attackers. It was a decisively powerful item. As
the movie progressed I watched as some small groups,
killing off most of their attacking opponents, grew strong
and powerful. Then, just as they would begin to feel they
had won the war, one of the survivors on the other side
would find an opponent's spent bullet and then the winning
side would get nearly wiped out all at once. This went on
and on; the attrition rate was terrible. Different groups, all
over the world, would grow strong and feel victorious only
then to be wiped out by the very thing which made them
victors.*

*After a while people began to realize that fighting would
accomplish absolutely nothing in the long run. As long as
they fought, their opponent—even if down to the last
man—could clobber them with one of their own spent
bullets. With this spent-bullet power universally available
to all, nobody could ever emerge as ultimate winner. As
soon as a group got close to that goal they would always
be demolished by one of their surviving opponents.
Domination of one nation by another had become
impossible.*

*In one scene I saw a large trailer with some military gear
in it. It was a combination of RADAR and computer equipment and all heavily guarded by machine guns. A woman
was attacking this trailer and she received a wound from a
machine gun bullet. She removed the bullet from her body
and it gave her the power. With her next shot she killed*

the machine gunner, climbed into the trailer and destroyed all the electronic equipment. The interior of the trailer caught fire and the woman, caught inside, died in it.

When people finally realized that nothing could be accomplished by fighting (as if it ever could!) they all decided to become peaceful and cooperate with one another. A scene appeared showing the United Nations organization. It had become very large and popular. People were distributing food, clothing, and tools to the underdeveloped peoples of the world. This would have made a happy ending to the film except for the last scene. It showed the Russians at it again. A lot of their soldiers were marching in a fancy drill team, all of which seemed to be showing off their military strength.

The spent bullet represents the psychological projection which always comes back at you. It behaves like a Karmic debt, like a boomerang! The belief system of the person doing the projecting is in denial of its ownership. Because of this blind spot, he or she is automatically vulnerable to manipulation by others.

$\mathcal{D}eath$ of the $\mathcal{N}eurosis$
Tribe LSD/Carbogen Session of 11-25-65

"When on Earth the flesh is lying,
let the winged soul be flying
to the joys of paradise."

— Poulenc, Stabat Mater, 1950
(Sacred Hymn)

Physiology of Carbogen

Carbogen is a mix of oxygen and carbon dioxide gases that is used for inhalation therapy in most hospitals. The air we breath consists of 21% oxygen and 0.03% carbon dioxide, with most of the balance being nitrogen. Carbogen consists of 80% oxygen and 20% carbon dioxide, give or take a few percent, depending upon the source. It contains no nitrogen and much more each of both oxygen and carbon dioxide than does air.

When a person suffocates or drowns, the resulting panic reaction is caused by a shift in brain chemistry. This panic does not derive from insufficient oxygen, however, but from excess carbon dioxide. So when one inhales carbogen the brain gets more than enough oxygen but at the same time it also gets an excess of carbon dioxide. This excess places the person in a state of mock suffocation. Everybody I have known to inhale carbogen experienced extreme fear and seemed to confront all the demons stored in his or her unconscious. This is the stuff of nightmares.

In psychotherapy, Carole used this breathing gas as a means of inducing one to confront these demons. If one has enough courage to hang in there with them and move toward them, as Carole often suggested, they lose their power over the patient. This is not unlike fearful figures in dreams that change their form and lose perceived power when confronted.[47]

In attendance at this particular Saturday Tribe session were two medical doctors, Larry and George. I had had some limited experience with carbogen so I knew how fearful one can get with only two or three breaths of the gas mix. Early in the day I watched Larry administer carbogen to George and was amazed. Larry instructed George to count down one number with each breath, starting with his age which was in the fifties. He spoke, loud enough to be heard through the mask, "fifty-three, (breath), fifty-two, (breath), fifty-one, (breath), etc," all the way down. I was unable to understand how anybody could remain lucid enough to do that for dozens of breaths. I hadn't been able to do so for more than one or two breaths before my fears took over and ran me. My respect for the psychic strength of George rose out of sight as I watched him.[48]

---

[47] This strategy, of confronting the fearful object, is remarkably similar to Temiar Indian teachings as reported by Richard Noone in *Search of the Dream People*, Wm Morrow & Co., 1972:
"The child must advance boldly against dream monsters, dream animals, and dream ghosts. If he defeats them, they become his slaves, but if he runs away, they will plague him until he seeks them out and fights them."

[48] Much later I came to realize that it was not a matter of present-time strength that allowed George to do this; it was a matter of past-time courage. Having already confronted that which Carbogen released in him, he had achieved a state of peace with himself under its influence.

Prologue

Out of death and out of the night came the vertical streamer. It flowed up and away from Earth as if repelled by the very matter from which it came. Our world is only a sphere of culture medium that grows life forms on its surface, out of the random stockpile of matter and energy. There is only one issue, one commitment: life or not-life. The organisms committed to not-life get stuck on the surface with gravity while the life-committed organisms have freedom. The sorting out is a noisy process with the screams of those left behind. The meaning of life is death and the meaning of death is life. Appearances are the reverse of reality; what is free to move out of its body is alive and what is stuck to cellular tissue dies with the tissue. No person can kill another person. You may fill a body with bullet holes but you cannot destroy the life-substance carried in the body. Killing another only serves to reduce the amount of life-substance in the killer.

This was an important session for me and Tribe for learning about reality and seeing meaning and order take form in the pasty mixture of all the elements of life.

The Lead-in

The authorities: Quentin for stash-dump; Charlie and Paula for the body of the session and myself for ceremony. Charlie, Carole's husband, was a man who spent half his time beside Carole helping to heal us and the other half of his time in need of healing himself. The session carried itself. Most of the plans that Charlie, Paula and I had made were dropped aside as the events picked up their own momentum. I had prepared several readings for the ceremony. In the doing, I cut out all but one (which was still too long). When 'boosted', that is under the influence of a psychedelic drug, people seem to flow and be psychically fluid. It becomes difficult or impossible to keep following the train of thought of something being read by another. A single passage from *The Prophet* is about as long as can be followed by the rational mind while the doors of perception of unconscious mind-material are open.

After the readings and candle lighting, I lay down with Ingrid and Quentin. We, together, let the process of opening up to the booster continue. We began to go places in our visual imagery that we described to one another. We viewed the same panorama as if we were actually traveling together. Our descriptions were almost, but not quite, identical—as if we were in the same place but were each seeing it through a different set of eyes or perhaps through a different porthole. It seemed to be a planet covered with sand or sand dunes. There were many beaches. Mostly we were high up, over water, traveling. I saw the sand dunes rapidly shifting as if seen with time-lapse photography. I also saw things awash on the beach coming and going with the waves. They were fragments of cloth with hand-embroidered patterns in color. I thought they were brought across the ocean from another culture. They looked like Scandinavian hand-sewn material such as is used in women's dresses or children's clothing. They looked all crinkly like seersucker and the colors had run a little. My first association was that they looked like counterfeit money looks, of poor quality, and I felt distrust of the people who had made them. Then I thought that perhaps I had some dishonest part of me which I was projecting onto the cloth. This was followed by another possibility that seemed more likely: the long immersion in the water had caused the appearance.

After a while Quentin began making noises of approaching some kind of strong emotion like ecstacy or something which feels shattering. These two emotions are similar for me. Carole and Dr. Larry brought the gas to him and he had two or three inhalations of gas. I lay with my head on his chest and felt that I was getting the effects of the drug on a low level.

The Main Event

The gas bottle was next passed to Ollie. I asked for, and was given the gas, next, while Quentin lay near me. With the first breath (I can't remember if I had three or four breaths altogether) I rapidly sank into part of my unconscious and saw a scene: I was suspended over a tile floor—from perhaps thirty feet high—in the patio of a building. I descended and the individual tiles became larger and I could see that each tile had an identical picture on it. I was feeling from the level of a child—I was carried back to my experience of early childhood. The pictures were either of my face as a child or else they were pictures of my father's face as it had looked to me during this part of my childhood. Possibly the pictures were first one and then the other—but they looked alike in some strange way. I could not tell which was which. There was no unique, separate identity for the two. Seeing these pictures I was swamped with intense negative feelings of self-hate and disgust. I felt myself going toward some kind of "death" and one level, the level of conscious intellect, wanted me to move toward the death. On another level—that of strong childhood narcissism*—I did not want the death. The narcissism was the stronger of the two. Instead of moving toward the death my path seemed to veer off into something intensely painful. I felt this pain while centered in the neurotic narcissistic part of my identity. This closeness to death induced another pain in me on yet another level of being: the observer level of consciousness that was losing out in the struggle and knew that it—the growth-directed level—would succumb if it lost the battle.

The level of pain was terrible and on the first trip the neurosis won out. After I came out of the gas (and equating death with pain) I said to Carole, "I don't want to die." She replied, "You'll have to die sometime Sweetie; don't you want to do it now while you are surrounded by those who love you and who will support you through the experience?" I said, "OK," and went into the gas a second time with the same results. Carole said I didn't have to do more at that session.

Freedom is a straight vertical line

I lay there on the floor sorting out the meaning of what I had experienced while someone else was having the gas. Some ugly things registered on my consciousness. I didn't want to look at them but I did so anyway. A recent but deep memory came into consciousness: I had, on some far off narcissistic level, wished Tracy (my mentally retarded daughter) to die instead of me. This intertwined with the awareness that at the same time my childhood narcissism had wanted my father to die instead of itself. However, since I wasn't clear about the separate identities of "father" and "me," the part of me that was my father had wanted the "I" part of me to die.[49] **I had wanted some other identity (i.e., aspect of my psyche projected onto someone else) to die instead of "me"—wherever I happened to be centered.** The intense pain came because I deflected the death onto another instead of willing it to come straight toward me. I had ducked taking responsibility for my own death experience.

The direction of death—I learned later when I finally broke through—seemed to be **vertical.** The other parts of myself—at the time represented by Tracy and my father—were across from me on the same horizontal plane. The line of authority or reality seemed to be the life-death

---

[49] I had been in a state of psychic dissociation with a fragmented personality. My psyche consisted of several entities and the conscious "I" was hopping around from one to another of them.

line—which was vertical—while all people on our level of existence were on the same horizontal plane.

Looking at this image on a larger scale, this plane becomes the surface of the Earth—a sphere—and the life-death line starts at the center of the planet and moves outward in any direction. It passes through the surface—always

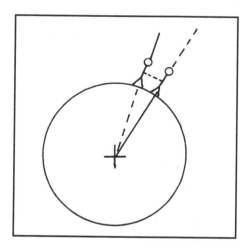

perpendicular to it—anywhere there is a human body. My wish to have someone else die instead of me put a little horizontal "kink" (toward another person) in my vertical line. Perhaps this is my attempt to splice half of someone else's line to half of mine; not only does it not work but in the attempt I get stuck because only half my vertical is left available to me. This kink prevented any vertical movement and this caused me to become "stuck" at the level of the Earth's surface instead of moving out of my body in the upward direction that is death. It was being "stuck" when there was so much pressure to move upward that seemed to cause the pain and screaming.

It was not the motion toward death that caused the pain but the avoidance of it!

This is the visual imagery conjured up by my unconscious mind that represents how narcissism, guilt, and finally, taking responsibility for my own destiny are woven into the fabric of life.

The Breakthrough

During the few minutes I lay resting I sorted this out and said to Carole, "I have another trip to make." Both she and Dr. Larry knew that I was hung up but had not suggested I have more of the gas. I felt that my knowledge of why I was hung up—if only in symbolic form—would enable me to get through the experience. I told them about the imagery and why I felt I had been stuck. Dr. Larry said, "When you were talking at stash-dump and spoke of Tracy that is just what went through my mind." So I was given more gas. This time I wanted my hands held.

During the resting period, I explained, I had felt close to a time (that must have been from a past life?) when I—a small boy—had crawled under a gas stove and gotten stuck and the gas was on or perhaps leaking. I had died or nearly died from breathing the gas. My arms had been caught under the stove and I was unable to move them. Thus I wanted my arms held to simulate this experience. Also, I felt they might fly around if not held.

This time I went into the gas and went straight toward the narcissistic part of me and—while my center stayed in the narcissism—I **did** experience the death of my ego. At first I fought it with all my strength but this time **I didn't shift the energy on to another person!** This tactic had become conscious and so could be consciously avoided. Being centered in my narcissism I felt the pain and fear of the narcissism approaching death. I felt filled to over-flowing with disgust and repulsion for the dishonesty of the narcissistic part—at its not taking responsibility for its own death and wanting another to die for it—but, since I *was* the narcissism the hatred was self-hate. Then something abruptly flipped. The self-hate became so strong and the pain so intense and the growth-directed part of me—that was outside the center of my identity at the time—felt so inadequate at not having been strong enough to take over, that I flipped into a strange state of letting go of the fight and giving up. This took place, however, while I remained centered in my narcissism! Then I was in the position of wanting to end the whole struggle but I felt I couldn't die because this had been what the struggle had been all about. Wasn't I giving up before I reached death? By this time Carole had removed the carbogen mask from my face I was screaming, "I want to die!" while feeling too unworthy and weak to do so. I was in a strange untenable position and the result was that I let go of **everything** and did have my death experience; I lost all consciousness and "it" took over and carried me through. I had been trying to do the dying but could not. When I released myself to it, the experience happened **to** me and not because **of** me. I feel that the death experience cannot take place unless control and power are relinquished and some larger but unseen power takes over to do the job. This sounds obvious but my neurosis had been pretty clever at convincing me that I had to do the dying, that I had to cause the death to take place through my own effort. Of course that was simply a devious means of avoiding the death. My neurosis was clever but not strong enough to prevail after I got the horizontal kink out of the vertical life-death line, that is, after I took responsibility for dying and stopped wishing someone else would do it for me.

Feeling weak and totally drained of energy as I regained consciousness, I asked Carole, "Did I die?" She smiled and said, affectionately, "Yes, you died." As I didn't recall parts of the experience I remained uncertain that I had made the breakthrough until a short time later. Tammy had watched me and mentioned that I had said, "I want to die." It was like suddenly remembering a dream I had shortly before. On hearing this I was able to recall the missing parts and knew that the experience had been complete. With this realization I felt better.

Having joined Tammy, I described to her some of the things that I had experienced. I began to feel a freedom that I had never felt before. I felt my psyche flow through time, space and other dimensions that we don't have names for. I felt that something extremely desirable had happened to me and felt an intense desire to find some means of retaining it, and if unable to retain it to capture something that would show how to return to it. I spent what seemed like two hours with my "computer" working flat out sorting out the meaning of the events and finding the order behind them. (We used the word *computer* as a label for the logical, rational part of the human mind, i.e., the neocortex. Remember, these events occurred well before personal computers existed.) Describing them to Tammy and getting her feedback helped enormously. I think that the first and strongest thing that came to me was that both our culture and I had a reversed view of the meaning of death. My new view of death held that death—the death of the body—has nothing to do with my earlier concept of death at all. When the cells fall apart and disintegrate is a happening quite apart from death. I felt that when I finally let go to the experience of death, all consciousness departed then something else took over. Some part of me left my body and moved vertically upward. This part of me (I will call it the *ethereal* for lack of a better term) returned when consciousness did. Meanwhile something about my narcissism that had been part of me did **not** return. Three things left, two returned, and responsibility replaced narcissism for me on that occasion.

The crucial moment for me came when I chose to take responsibility for my death-wish for another. That is, when I brought it to consciousness and, seeing it, withdrew it from others. In doing so I straightened out the kink in my life-death line that allowed my vertical motion.

This new perspective on death was that moving out of the body and upward is not death at all as it is usually thought of. This is not to be confused with the near-death experience of the **body** described by Elizabeth Kübler-Ross and others. My experience was the death of the **neurosis,** where leaving the body, paradoxically, is a necessary step for growth, and hence, is life sustaining. Staying in the body and clinging to consciousness when it is time to die is, again paradoxically, what real spiritual death is. If this happens when the body is destroyed, then the psyche stays stuck in the matter that was the body and does not move up the vertical line to the Great Spirit. The neurosis (for lack of a better word) seems to be unable to move upward and is dependent upon staying with the cells and tissue for survival. This part is mortal. During the gas/death experience the mortal part, as usual, tries to draw my consciousness into **its** space so the movement up and out will not take place. The rule is, consciousness will defend whatever space it occupies at the time. This "neurosis" part of me may be operationally defined in this analogy as the part that cannot move out of the body. The reason it cannot move is that each "cell" of the neurosis (the ethereal equivalent of a cell) has something in it analogous to a chromosome: something with pattern or form that characterizes its essential quality. This form in the "neurosis' ethereal cell" is the kink—a horizontal kink in the vertical line which is the line of life/death. The kink is created by deflecting responsibility on to another.

The result of my pointing my problems at someone else instead of toward my own Godliness—my higher spiritual authority—for resolution, is that it leaves me mired in my painful neurotic responses.

If you are not willing to die, you don't get to.
My belief is that the culturally established notion that life is inherent in cellular tissue is only partly correct. Life

appears here as something that gets its start in a body of cells much as a yeast culture may start and grow in a test tube. The people on our planet appear to me to be similar to a culture of cells in the Petri dish but on a larger scale. The origin of life in the body certainly seems to be connected with bio-tissue. After it is well established there I now, however, question whether tissue is necessary for the continued existence of the consciousness we associate with life. Indeed, when the time comes for the natural death of the body that stuff that I call life (**soul** is probably a better word) continues to grow and develop. It moves upward, away from the planet's surface, and out of the Petri dish of incubation. The function of the planet seems to be twofold: First, it is a starting place for the origin of life (in tissue). Second, it acts as a selection filter for sorting out the kink-free ethereal cells from those that are kinked. During a natural death the first moves up and away from the tissue and the second stays behind. It is as if the surface of the earth is covered with something like a metal screen (acting as a sieve) through which nothing with a horizontal kink can pass. If life collects in tissue, on the planet, and later moves off its surface into ethereal space (at tissue death), then the part that is responsible for its life and death must be separated from that which develops on the planet that is kinked. Here I mean that part that is inclined to duck its responsibility toward its own death and would have another die in its place. Perhaps this part, stuck on Earth, is manifest in all of us who are still reincarnating?

During the years of my therapy and with Tribe, I began to value certain things: relationships, love, creativity, openness, life, explorations of the unconsciousness, etc. I had never been able to rank these in value, however, or place them in a hierarchy. Following my death experience under carbogen I became convinced that the highest value of them all is **life.** I spoke of this to Carole at the conclusion of Tribe session. After all, without life we would not have any other values.

Jesus died as an act of love for his fellow humans but, in so doing, he taught (by example) the unreal association that life may be sacrificed in the service of love. It became clear to me that love can effect life-destructive events and so love, even, must be ranked below life on the hierarchy of values. I don't mean life is to be chosen at the expense of love, but I struggle with the idea that Jesus chose love at the expense of life. When God gave his only begotten son so the rest of us can have everlasting life and when people equate life **only** with cellular tissue an incorrect conclusion is reached: "I can achieve **tissue** immortality and therefore should seek to do so." For those who read scripture this way something got lost in translation here. My view is that the death of the body releases the spirit to be **born** into its next existence whatever that may be. Thus death and birth are two sides of the same coin.

When I walked into this session the constellation formed by the elements of my neurotic mind resembled that of Narcissus viewing his image in the water. I describe much of my experience in terms of this narcissism. Perhaps this was because I simply responded from my particular hang-up or perhaps it was because one's narcissism is universally elicited by carbogen. I have no way of telling which. To me, arising from this session, narcissism is exemplified by an unconscious expression of a person's desire for another's death when the other causes or appears to cause some problem. This other person may be mother saying to child, "You may **not** have any more candy," or it may be the total stranger who has just run into your car and creased your fender. The real problem is internal, of course, but gets projected on the person who is perceived to cause it. This projection of the problem and the accompanying piece of death-wish directed toward another person is the horizontal kink in the otherwise vertical life-death line. It is there because if the person didn't exist (i.e., were dead) the perceived problem would not exist. The kink is horizontal because matter—cells, tissue, body—is limited by time, space and gravity. These keep all bodies on the horizontal surface so that any two people in relationship are horizontally opposed to one another. No two people can be in the same place at the same time. So, when a problem develops there are two ways to cope: One may solve it by **either** making an internal adjustment and then by taking appropriate external action, **or** one can project the problem onto someone else resulting in a little death-wish for that other person, even though the problem may eventually be resolved by appropriate external action. Now, if the solution is attempted by actual destruction of the object of the projection—by murder to use the most extreme example—the ethereal cells of the murderer are changed and kinked because the act of murder is a demonstration of destructive irresponsibility. I feel that we inherit from our past lives a residue of these kinks from all the destructive acts we have done. The murders, the acts of physical violence and the molestations are all attempts to shift responsibility of death onto another, and kinked ethereal cells result. We can, according to this belief system, unkink them and clean up our karma by re-living the acts of past lives in structured, life-directed, consciousness-inducing situations such as, for example, group therapy.

Grist for today's mill

When I was on my way to Albany with my daughter Tracy, the Friday morning preceding this session, I looked at her on the way to the car. I thought to myself, consciously, "If she were to die I wouldn't have to do these things that I don't want to do." Driving her to her school, 150 miles away, and doing the rest of the things that have to be done by me for Tracy, for whom I am responsible, prevents me from doing other things that I would rather be doing. Thus, I pictured her as a problem; that is, I had projected the problem onto her and wished her dead.

Acts of violence that harm people physically cause these kinks. I now see, with impact, the meaning and reason we in Tribe have put so much stress on not hurting anybody physically. What we have been doing is getting our kinks straightened as we apply what we learn in therapy. What kinks we have from our past lives (and from past-time acts perpetrated earlier in our present lives **if we learn from them**) are small compared to those we acquire in perpetrating acts of destruction in present time. It does no good to work out the past hang-ups only to negate all that work by later slugging, perhaps one's therapist, and setting in a kink that is bigger than the sum of all those undone. Just why we get possessed with the kinks of past lives I don't understand but it certainly is parallel to the Karma concepts from Hinduism.

A Cosmic Key

Discussing the session with Tammy I described the key I had seen in my visual imagery. What it meant to me, I explained, was that we have been given some kind of "key" by other entities. Whether those who left it came from some other planet or from this one I don't know. It really doesn't matter, for when the spirit of a creature is separated from its material body, it is indistinguishable from the spirit of non-human beings whom we would describe as "alien." This key was, I felt sure, left to us many eons ago. Perhaps it exists somewhere deep in the collective unconscious or in the Akashic Records*? I saw it long enough to write this report describing events that excited me with a feeling of revelation. All I have seen during this session puts the work the Tribe has been doing for years in a new perspective. A new kind of elegant order to all our work has taken shape.

When I saw the key I also saw the picture seen in magazine advertisements of the Rosicrucian society. In this picture is a key (plus a pyramid) and the ad addresses the "secrets of life" left to us by the "ancients." When this came up and I described it to Tammy I felt an overwhelming love from the entities who left us this key. They have long since moved on toward their destinies, whatever they may be, and may never see or meet us. They left the key with absolute unconditional love. Their leaving something like this for us and moving on, never to see us, deeply moved me. There seems to be great wisdom in the way the key has been left. To reach the key, an individual must explore his or her unconscious and learn how they tie in with the collective unconscious, which means that all the neurotic and non-life oriented parts of the person must be worked through and resolved. The path to **wholeness** must be undertaken. Only then can the box containing the key be approached. There is elegance in this means of selecting only those who are dedicated to life and reality and rejecting those who are dedicated to a reality-as-they-would-like-it-to-be rather than the Truth.

I sought Quentin, our mathematician, specifically for discussion of this. In mathematics, a proof or solution that is ingenious and simple and straight to the point with an absence of frills is termed "elegant." This is just how the key has been left to us, with cosmic elegance. The elegant simplicity of the pattern and its meaning broke me into tears as I described it to Quentin.

This "key" feels like something that each individual must find for himself; each person must go all the way through his/her personal unconscious to reach it, but the more we, as individuals, approach our own key and learn about the path, the easier and faster will be the path of the others in Tribe to his or her personal key.

Psychic massage

Just after my last carbogen scene, and before I began talking about my gas experience with Tammy, I sat behind her and put my hands on her temples. We sat thus for perhaps ten or fifteen minutes in a meditative state and neither moving nor speaking. Our bodily interface, the zones of contact between my hands and her head, became tactually transparent; we fused. Our etheric bodies had become one body. I was able to move my etheric hands past the interface, through our skins, and into Tammy's etheric body. Then I began doing what I can only describe as "pulling out splinters of things." The splinters were large, perhaps the equivalent of several non-inches but shorter than a non-foot. As this took place I saw Tammy become more relaxed and fluid. Following this activity, when we finally moved into a new position, Tammy said she felt my hands were at the base of her brain and doing "something good." It felt to me that this kind of healing was what masseur Zach was striving to do when I had my first massage from him several weeks before. Zach, a chiropractic doctor, and I had become backpacking buddies and, later on, he taught me the art of Swedish massage. I felt that his hands did some deep healing on my ethereal body with his first massage. With the most recent one I received from him, the Friday before my carbogen session, however, he seemed to give only a normal massage and his hands didn't have the same internal sorting-out quality they had earlier.

Here, it seemed to me, was another fascinating aspect of this natural selection device. I felt that the ability to move one's ethereal body through space already occupied by another's physical body would embody great power for either good or evil. The selection factor that places this power into only those hands that will be used creatively is this: before one's ethereal hands can enter another's ethereal body they must first be able to freely move **out** of the massager's ethereal body. In order for this to happen, however, there must be no horizontal kinks just as they must be absent for a person to leave the body during a bodily death experience. With an absence of kinks it is a foregone conclusion that the hands entering another's ethereal body will be used responsibility and constructively. The selection factor is that this ability is naturally denied the irresponsible person, who, stuck in the physical body by the horizontal kink of irresponsibility, cannot move in this domain. What a gift, I thought, to have bestowed on me the ability for this healing work. This must be the result of the clarity I reached upon giving up the life of my neurotic narcissism.

Another thing I talked about with Tammy was my father. In his old age he had told me many of his experiences and conclusions. I suggested he write a book and share his wisdom. He said that he was totally pessimistic about how the world was going to blow itself up, and what was the use of his writing a book? Under the carbogen I saw him as a person already dead; I saw his ethereal body as a pile of ashes even though his physical body is still living. I cried from the grief of knowing of the death of a parent. I said to Tammy, "He is already dead and I can't do anything for him." I saw an image of the Arc de Triomphe in Paris and I saw the "eternal flame" that burns under it but the flame had gone out and there was nothing but a square pile of ashes as a stand-in symbol for my father. This imagery came from my knowledge of his history: He fought in World War I in France. Later I decided that perhaps there is some chance for him but the only thing I can do is show him how and where I am. If he should take hope from seeing my freedom then perhaps he will move out of his pile of ashes. I felt that he was terribly hung-up in his cells and unable to move toward real extra-cellular life because some soldiers, attempting to follow his orders, were killed in the process. I think he carried guilt over this all the rest of his life.

More symbology that I saw but that is difficult to describe: All the molecules of my body were represented by a complicated set of lines that joined at many places. I felt that—before my carbogen death experience—all the empty spaces between the rods and nodes were filled with something like mud or clay. Afterward all the mud had dropped away and now there remained only the rods and nodes. The absence of the clay allowed my ethereal body to move through all the dimensions at will. I thought of the feeling I had a week or two ago when, as I had described to Tribe, I felt myself encumbered by my body and cells as I did when in SCUBA costume and under water.[50] Now, I felt free of any encumbrance to my body. I was in a 'state of grace' with an indescribable sense of freedom.

A freeing question
When I sat with Tammy I felt not able to completely open to her and, examining this, I asked myself:

---

[50] Wearing a thick, custom-fitted, foam rubber suit that squeezes the body, carrying all that hardware strapped to the body, looking through a tunnel-vision faceplate and breathing air through a pressure valve that requires a hard pull from one's diaphragm to yield air, all contribute to activate any latent claustrophobia.

"At what times and under what conditions do I have little unconscious or conscious death wishes for her?"[51]

As I thought about this I realized that the one time this occurred was when I saw or was with another sexually attractive woman with whom I wanted to make love. My perceived problem—not able to have sex with the woman—not getting what I wanted—was projected onto Tammy and my unconscious thought was ". . . if Tammy were dead I would not have this problem." Of course the thought of wishing Tammy, my wife, dead was unacceptable[52] and so had remained in my unconscious

---

[51] As narcissism is a childish state, so is the form of this "death wish." According to Joan Grant, writing in *Many Lifetimes*,
"Death to healthy children means, "to go somewhere else," so what is more natural than that they should wish that an irksome member of the household, who has refused to take hints that his absence would be a welcome relief, should depart by dying?"

[52] James Michener writes on this delimma in *Tales of the South Pacific*. During WWII an American officer named Bus, dating a native girl named Latouche, completely charmed her:

"Oh Bus!", she cried, "I wish you not married. I wish my husban' he dead. You and I we get married..."
"Latouche!" I whispered. "For God's sake, don't talk like that."
"Why not? I wish my husban' he dead up there in the hills. Then everything all right. I marry some nice American.
"Stop it!"
"Whatsomatter, Bus? You no wish your wife she dead sometime?"
"It's not funny, Latouche!" I protested. My forehead was wet.
"I not say it funny," she mused, quietly buttoning her dress. "I talk very serious. When you kissing me? When you taking my dress off? I s'pose you never wish your wife dead?"
I felt very funny inside. You know how it is. You're out in the islands. You have a wife, but you don't have a wife. *Sometimes the idea flashes through your head... Without your thinking it, understand. And you draw back in horror. "What*

mind. When I saw what it was, a death-oriented kink, the thing lifted from me and I was then able to open up. One "splinter" I removed from her ethereal brain was connected with my recently brought-to-consciousness death-wish. This particular one was the easiest to remove. Others were more difficult and some I couldn't touch at all. I feel I was able to work on ones that were appropriate for me to act on and the rest were simply inaccessible to me. It is as though the authority to reach them is a function of the depth of my commitment to accepting responsibility for the shadow* side, the dark side, of my psyche.

At the end of the day, as I hugged or chatted with each person in Tribe, I asked myself, **"In what ways have I ever wished this person dead?"** A quick search of my historical memory with him or her followed. With some, I found a place; with others I did not. In general, it seemed that when there is a person with whom I have a neurotic problem there is a little death-wish. Deliberately looking for these past time wishes serves to bring them to consciousness. **Assuming responsibility for their existence allows them to surface to conscious awareness.** Only then do I have the freedom to do something about their acts of creation. Instead of running me, as they had in the past, I can now see what my unconscious motives are and figure out how I want to change. It is an act of taking responsibility for my hostility. Carl Jung describes the *autonomous complex* as an unconscious psychic entity that, because the conscious person has denied its existence, is able to run the person's life. These complexes lose their autonomy and hence their power when brought to consciousness. As I hugged my friends, one by one, and

---

in hell am I saying? What kind of man am I, anyway?"
The italics are mine, not Michener's. Note the inherent unacceptability of the thought.

examined my death-wishes for them, I broke out of
whatever block these had formed in me. I felt myself more
able to flow and relate with and love that person.
Following that, taking responsibility for it—withdrawing
the projected energy out of the other person—is immediately helpful in the growth process. Carole defines
love as **the absence of barriers.** Here I was sequentially
bringing to consciousness barriers to my friends, removing
them, and feeling the love expand. The cause-and-effect
demonstrated by this was dramatic. The lesson I learned
was to prove most helpful to me:

**The mere knowledge of what to look for can bring a
neurotic hook into consciousness!**

Martyrs are suicidal ham actors

With this new perspective I saw the martyr in a new light.
His act of destroying his own body, whether actively or by
passively allowing others to do it, even done in the name of
"saving" others, remains an irresponsible act. Whether he
wishes another dead or allows himself to die for another, a
kink in the vertical line to the Great Spirit is created. This
orientation causes him to become stuck in his tissue and not
ascend upward with his bodily death. In so doing he
"saves" neither himself nor anyone else. He only teaches,
by his action, that death is of higher value than life—a
false equation. Placing physical life and death in a
hierarchical value system makes as much sense as saying
that the force of gravity is "better than" the force of mag-
netism. To struggle to avoid the natural death of the body
is just as counterproductive as is suicide which is a struggle
to avoid natural life. If **we** didn't choose our bodies and
life-dramas, then who did? In making this choice we made
an agreement to hang in there with the body and use it for
growth and enlightenment. To me, the martyr is selling the
people "for whom he died" a bill of goods: death is a
higher order or more noble than life (or it could just as well

be vice versa). Martyrdom, as I see it, is something inherently dishonest. To me, this lie was neurotic crap which makes it that much more difficult for others to either grow or die naturally. This makes martyrdom an act of destruction to others—a strange concept to me but only, perhaps, because it is new. It leaves me with a contradiction. In Jesus' case, it is clear that he knew what he was doing when he raked over the money-lenders; he knew that the establishment would come down on him. He went ahead and created his own martyrdom. My conflict is that I believe Jesus was a totally loving person, yet his martyrdom was an unloving act. There must be something missing from my picture of this event.

Epilogue

At the beginning of this report I described how Dr. George had been able to inhale dozens of breaths of carbogen and appear to remain comfortable and unmoved. My amazement came from my not knowing that the demons residing in one's unconscious mind, once faced and confronted, vanish like smoke. I had assumed that he was a man of great courage to be able to continue counting in the face of all those frightening demons. I now know that he had already confronted his and, for him, they were no more. I had an opportunity to inhale carbogen during 1974, three years after I left Carole's therapy. I was amazed and gratified at how different the experience was for me than my earlier one. I was totally comfortable, clearheaded and at peace with myself under the gas. I felt no panic or fear and lay completely relaxed for several minutes. I finally removed the mask and handed it to the doctor whose gas I was breathing because I didn't want to empty his gas bottle! Certainly it was carbogen I had been breathing because I watched my friend Marco, naive to breathing carbogen, breathe from the same bottle. He went into a typical panic state almost immediately. On his third or fourth breath, he sat up and yanked the mask off with great urgency and—for a few seconds until he got his bearings—had to have his flailing arms restrained.

This observation reinforced my belief that I had, indeed, confronted and conquered all the fears that can be induced by this gas mixture.

On Mandala Symbology

Much of the energy which produced this book has come from visual imagery, which is one of my strongest gifts. As an addendum to the session of Birth/Rebirth, here is a description of the ubiquitous **cross.** The visual imagery I encountered under carbogen, with the horizontal and vertical axes, (along with much thought about it) yielded this interpretation of our most highly emotionally charged symbol:

The Christian cross is a distorted member of the mandala family. The mandala has, typically, strong symmetry.[53] Usually the field is quartered although it may be divided, radially, into anywhere from three to sixteen parts. In the quartered mandala the dividing lines are usually horizontal and vertical. The intersection of these lines is the center of the figure. Cross-hairs. Perfect balance. Peace. Wholeness. All these are there.

The words *horizontal* and *horizon* are derived from a common root. Our large planet (large relative to our bodies) and its gravitational force configures our horizon.

---

[53] *Mandala* is sanskrit for *Magic Circle.*

On this symbol, Jung offers, on page 335 of, *Memories, Dreams, Reflections,* 1961, "The mandala is an archetypal image whose occurrence is attested throughout the ages. It signifies the wholeness of the self."

He then defines *Disturbed Mandala,* on page 396 as, "Any form that deviates from the circle, square, or equal-armed cross . . ."

Stand erect and look at the horizon sweeping from your left
to your right. Hang a carpenter's plumb line from your
outstretched arm. It makes a vertical line exactly
perpendicular to your horizon—a perfect mandala. This is
the core and archetypical form of all mandalas. It is created out of the laws of physics which formed our planet and
the planet's inherent forces which influence our lives.

Carl Jung formulated his theory of the collective
unconscious from the study of widely diverse and disparate
cultures throughout history. People of many of these
cultures created artistic symbols for the most part identical
to symbols from other cultures. There is no historical
evidence that cross-cultural communication ever took place
between many of them. One of the most pervasive of these
symbols is the mandala. It appears, in many forms, in
virtually all cultures—the most isolated as well as frequently melded ones. It was this absence of any tangible,
physical, historical cross-cultural links in consciousness that
led Jung to his hypothesis: that if there are no links in consciousness to explain the artistic anomaly then there must
be a cross-cultural link outside consciousness, hence the
collective unconscious. Jung also points out that mentally
unbalanced and institutionalized people draw, not
infrequently, mandala figures. He explains that these
people have a spontaneous drive toward mental stability
which is expressed and aided by these mandala drawings.

To me the horizontal line represents humanity. It
represents the link one person has to another. It is
visualized as the space through which people talk to one
another or by the telephone wire connecting them. It
represents equality. The two people at the ends of the
horizontal link are at the same elevation with no ranking or
hierarchy. It represents my relationship with other people.

The vertical line represents my link with God, the Great
Spirit, the collective unconscious. I am always at the
Earth-surface of this line. This spiritual line starts at the
core of Earth and rises vertically, one through each of us,
threading its way through the seven chakras of the body.
When you and I stand near each other our vertical spiritual
lines appear parallel. It is our tiny size compared to
Earth's that creates this illusion. Parallel lines never meet.
Our spirit lines meet at the Earth's center at one end and
meet God at the other end. Both ends meet. This reflects
God as infinity, that which is overwhelming. In my
imagery, the vastness of space is too overwhelming to
comprehend. Its vastness represents, again, God's infinite
nature.

The mandala is reflected in the compass rose, four perfect
quarters and two (or four) lines of symmetry, North-South
and East-West. No line, of these four, is longer or shorter
than any other. No quarter has more or less area than any
other. Both balance and symmetry are perfect. To test
whether a figure has symmetry about an axis, lay it on a
flat surface. Then place a mirror's edge on its surface on
one of the lines of symmetry, with the mirror perpendicular
to the surface of the figure. The reflection must be
identical with that which it conceals for symmetry to exist.
If the mirror itself were invisible the figure would not
change; you would not be able to tell if the mirror were
present or not.

The inherent beauty of the mandala's perfect symmetry
across two axes is lost with the Christian cross. One arm is
longer than the rest. It is the bottom arm representing man
in the Man-God, or woman in the Woman-God relationship.
It is bigger than the arm representing God. It is longer because it had to be stuck in the ground deep enough to
support the weight of Jesus. The sado-masochistic under-
pinning of the structure of Judeo-Christianity has unbal-

anced the mandala of relationships. No longer are we, this symbol says, equal to each other and to God. Jesus, in choosing to allow his execution, and those who murdered him, created so much collective guilt that it stretched out the lower arm of their mandala for the rest of time. From the crucifixion onward, we have been driven into the ground by our now distorted image of God. We have lost something important here. I think we need to restore symmetry to our cross. My tendency is to study all religions. The Eastern ones have symmetrical crosses, balanced mandalas. Perhaps this is because, unlike Judaism, Christianity, and Islam, they have **no martyrs** in their histories?

$\mathcal{A}$ Capsule $\mathcal{I}$mplanted in $\mathcal{M}$y $\mathcal{B}$ody

Dream of 5-8-67

In this dream I found myself in contact with agencies from another level of existence. They were not subject to any of the limitations imposed upon us by space and time. (We have these limitations because we live in material bodies.) I didn't meet them directly or individually but was able to see some of the things which, by not being subject to our limitations, they were capable of doing. They were fantastic things, specifics of which I don't remember except for one: directly changing the DNA code of a person's cells.

Next I saw what was some kind of "implant" which they put in certain people. It looked in size and shape like a gelatin capsule and was made of silver colored metal. This device was implanted in a person's right shoulder, just below the clavicle, through an opening made through the front surface of the shoulder. One of the agencies told me that the operation left a very slight indentation on the front surface of a person's shoulder—the only visible sign of the operation. I looked at my right shoulder and saw a slight indentation but, more visible than that, was a small patch of pink skin, about 1/4" in diameter, just where the indentation was. This was new skin grown over the spot where the operation was done. This pinkness would disappear in a few weeks as is usual with small wounds. I had seen this pink spot previously, in the dream sequence, but had thought nothing of it; perhaps it didn't register on my consciousness. I knew, then, that one of the devices had been implanted in me.

Inside the implant capsule, I knew, was a fantastic amount of things which functioned like electronic circuitry but were many times more sophisticated than anything humans have done or even dreamed of. I was told one specific thing about my capsule: It contained a calendar, a "clock" of some kind that operated independent of bodily functions. This calendar could tell what day of the week it was and transmit this information back to the alien agencies. It was programmed only to be concerned with Mondays, sending a signal on that day and ignoring the rest. I thought it must sense the planet's circadian cycle and tell the day of week by counting. In the dream I tried to think of the possible significance of Mondays and could only postulate that due to a calendar change many years ago what we now call Monday used to be Sunday. I must have felt that Sunday signified the end of the week and they wanted a synchronizing signal each week.

My feelings about the capsule in my body were ambivalent. I met several humans, very creative people, tops in their fields, from all over the Earth, and they all had implants like mine. My implant placed me in flattering company. Furthermore, all these people seemed to be in contact with the alien agencies. My ambivalence was because I didn't know the function of the capsule. Was it a device the agencies would use to control me? Was it a "bug" they would use to tune in on me and learn what I was doing? I wasn't sure.

I woke up then and immediately knew why Mondays had been chosen—it was connected with the Monday Tribe meetings. This weekly routine had become engraved into my life. I also knew that the implant was not a "bug." The agencies didn't need any. Being not limited by time or space they could see any part of my life at any time if they so chose. I also knew it was not a control device; the agencies are not interested in any control over us. We are here to learn for ourselves and, if learning does not take place, the inherent program of our physical existence will control the outcome for better or worse. These agencies don't have to control me; such doesn't even interest them.

I then felt that the capsule was like an analog of a "graduation gift" and I felt proud to have been selected for it. Its function now seemed like something which can give those who have it information about different levels of reality for which we have, normally, no receptors in our bodies. Perhaps it enables me to communicate with the agencies when in need of help?

The presence of my implant was connected with my coming under legitimate authority. The years of hard work and learning to discriminate between valid and invalid authority allowed me to come under the valid authority of the agencies. In my particular life, this learning was intimately connected with my membership in the Monday Tribe and this is why the thing sends out a signal every Monday.

The other people given implants each had learned to discriminate between valid and invalid authority in their own ways. Their implants are not Monday-programmed but are programmed in other ways. Their programming reflected some aspect of their lives which enabled this learning to take place. All these people had one thing in common: besides being creative and successful they were highly diversified and were involved in many fields.

Author's note:
Between the occurrence of this dream and the writing of this book, 23 years later, a few best selling books have appeared about people claiming to have been abducted by UFO creatures. One of their claims is that they involuntarily underwent implant surgery in their shoulders, leaving small pink, dimpled scars. I have no explanation regarding the apparent congruence of this description with my earlier dream except to suggest that both stories came from the same source: our collective unconscious mind.

Acceptance of the Irrational
Tribe LSD Session of 5-30-67

By this time, Tammy and I were estranged to the extent
that she was now in a committed relationship with Willard
and I was spending my nights alone. We met Willard
through Carole, the woman we had hired to, hopefully, heal
our marriage. After all our years of struggle together to
grow beyond the strife we created for one another, in the
end we failed. I lost Tammy to another of my
psychotherapist's patients. What remained of my
relationship with Tammy revolved mostly around Thea, our
daughter. My meager visitation "rights" did in no way
convince me that I still had a daughter in my life. Like
what remained of my relationship with Tammy, what was
left of my relationship with Thea was, I felt, little more
than an empty shell.

It was a very sad time in my life. In terms of my
psychotherapy I see, in hindsight, that this would have been
the appropriate time for me to terminate my treatment. The
very thing that drew me to therapy, the threat I felt to my
marriage relationship, was now moot. However, in terms
of the emotional state I was in, following the loss of my
wife and child, I very much needed the emotional support
of Tribe, my emotional family. And so I stayed on,
working my way through life one day at a time; I couldn't
see any definitive future ahead.

The Session Report
There was very little talk during this session relative to
previous ones. This report is therefore a long one to cover

what was not discussed during the session itself. The stash-dump period revealed no gross problems except for Frank, who refused to see any point to learning; he never mentioned the word *learning* during his stash-dump. He was uptight through both the session and the free-swinging time afterward. I saw no sign of movement on his face and he had the "left out" expression of a small boy just on the edge of sulking but too passive to move out of it. Dedication to not feeling good is its own punishment.

The focus for this session was on three things:

First was that together we made a three-tiered universal commitment: A) to feel what we were at the time, B) to totally express the feeling, if appropriate, and, C) to ask for help if needed.

At the beginning when we made this commitment I saw no particular significance to it but later, during the psychic movement, it became a real anchor for me. Always, if in doubt about something taking place in me (or perceived in another), I would go back to the anchor: "What am I feeling?" Oh, yeah . . . then feel it totally from the tips of my toes to the top of my scalp and with all of my cells vibrating from that feeling.

The **second** was the theme for the day: the acceptance of the irrational. Learning about this has simplified my life and I am glad for it. Most of the feelings I had were baffling—way beyond the reach of my understanding—and so I would accept the irrationality of the feeling and go ahead and feel it without questioning what it meant or censoring it.

The **third** item in focus came from our discussion of being *both* father and son and with this one I started the session: in imagination I became both father protecting son and the protected son. I became a figure about my actual age (really, in a sense, ageless), standing in a forest wearing clothing like someone from a Robin Hood novel, deerskin and peaked hat with a bow slung over my shoulder. The son was dressed in similar clothing and about five years old. I was able to feel the role of father but not that of son. Then I felt the presence of a third figure, the father's father, and I easily fitted into the role of this man's son. All this took place in about fifteen minutes.

I looked around the circle and felt isolated as I saw the people in their respective committed relationships together: Quentin/Jane, Tammy/Willard, and Charlie/Carole. I wondered if I was feeling sorry for myself. If so it felt inappropriate. Then what to do and what does the feeling of isolation mean in the here and now? I felt that what I needed and wanted from a relationship with a woman was some kind of psychic nourishment. I thought I would like to become, here, both the son and the **mother** in the same way as I became father and son. Then perhaps I can learn to nourish myself? I became both as I (son) suckled and I (mother) nourished. Mother looked like a fat Jewish mamma and the son changed to a small seedling which had just emerged from the soil. I was caught between overprotecting the seedling from the hostile forces of the world and allowing the sunlight in. The overprotection was two-edged:

　　　1) I wanted to believe that only I could provide the nourishment and therefore the sunlight wasn't essential, and

　　　2) I wanted to protect the seedling from strong winds which really could harm it.

Cutting off sunshine, however, means death to the young plant so I went through cycles of opening and closing my protective arms around the plant. Part of my mind knew that overprotection would kill the plant but Mamma was neurotically dependent upon the growth of the son and could not allow a greater nourishment in from outside the relationship. With this imagery I realized that something was wrong with the concept of self-nourishment. I put the computer to work on it and concluded that I was making a difficult task out of something which should be completely natural and spontaneous. I cannot nourish myself—only the Earth and the Sun can do that, and if I open myself to these the nourishment will be natural and automatic, just as experienced by a flower.

Carole, upon hearing my description of this, suggested that I feel disconnected from nature and had me look out the window at the green things. This felt good but I knew I needed more, so I decided to do more backpacking in the wilderness that summer. Carole changed the music and lay on top of me. I assumed she sensed a need in me and wanted to feel it out. I was glad to have her at that time to flow with. Then the start of strange, irrational feelings came to me. Almost as soon as she came to me I felt a surge of anger toward Carole. My computer went into high gear: Why? What was it? In the past it has always meant there was something I should explore. Should I verbalize this feeling? Wasn't sure. Then my commitment hit me and I knew that this edge of hostility, which I couldn't understand, was something I should open myself to and feel fully. When I did so I felt a huge rush of psychic movement. This felt right and I then knew that as long as the psychic work and flow was going without getting stuck it wasn't necessary to verbalize any of it. Verbalization would only stop the flow.

So—angry I felt and became to the core. In fantasy I screamed at Carole and tore her to shreds. I pounded and pummelled her and soon the hostility was gone. (All this with Carole lying on me.) It was instantly replaced by a little piece of some other feeling which at first I neatly tucked into one of my big toes where it would be out of sight. Again my commitment came into focus and I said, "Ah-ha! What is **that** feeling?" I pulled it out of my toe and saw what it was: GUILT. Understanding what it meant didn't matter any more. I took the guilt and wrapped it around myself and rolled in it until all my cells vibrated with it. It was a rather hideous experience, by the way. About that time I was able to generalize that the secret of the day for me was to feel, totally, whatever floated into my feelers. Once the guilt feeling was accepted totally it floated away and was, again, immediately replaced by another feeling which sank into my right middle toe. Upon pulling it out and examining it I found it was sexual desire for Carole. OK, I rolled in **that** and in fantasy said to her, "Carole, I want to fuck you," while I felt both the sexuality and the greed/desire. When this reached totality I had an insight about it. It was not Carole I desired, it was my mother! I had carried this residue of sex desire for years but had not allowed the feeling to consciousness because of the guilt which had been implanted in me concerning incest. With this insight the sexual feeling drifted off.

Then, and only then, was I free to feel the real Carole. She had been on my body for perhaps fifteen minutes. Half this time I did the feeling things with my emotional baggage and half I simply felt the warm, loving bond with her.

After changing music again, Carole lay between Charlie and me, and this three-way psychic fusing began its work. Wagner was playing, which usually carries me, on a high cloud of transcendence, to a unity experience, but on this occasion it happened only briefly. I went through a feeling of grief which passed shortly. The vigilant focus I maintained on totally feeling what I was at the moment seemed to keep me grounded from the cosmic. There is nothing, absolutely nothing, which feels as meaningful and fulfilling to me as the experience of cosmic unity. This experience is also something over which I have no control—it is given to me by some other. I felt disappointed as I realized the focus on total feeling seemed to be keeping me grounded except for a brief glimpse; I knew our commitment wasn't an arbitrary thing and there was a reason for it all, so I didn't get hung up about it. I don't know how the cosmic experience is meted out to people but I felt sure it was given in absolutely appropriate amounts, however irrational it may appear to us mortals, so I didn't question it.

Eventually I will learn, I don't doubt, how to keep totally immersed in my feelings and still reach the cosmic. Obviously I still have work to do before I am ready for that. The experience of staying totally, one hundred percent, in tune with my irrational (or otherwise) feelings is new to me. I need more familiarity with the full present-time task of feeling in harmony with the irrational to lift clear of the ground. It reminds me of learning to drive a car. In the beginning, I couldn't even crank the window up or down while attempting to cope with all the controls, etc.

Another feeling drifted in, hostility to the point of extreme desire to violently destroy. Feeling confident that my commitment to not hurting anybody, physically, was solid, I allowed this new feeling. I became the essence of embodied hostility but without any of its action. My body grew, in my imagination, sharp and jagged. There grew giant rose thorns and knives out of all my joints. Elbows, knuckles, toes, and knees were all armed to the teeth. My body had no bones, muscles or flesh. It was a total body of hostile violence. I was astonished that I had all that in me. In fantasy I ripped and shredded Charlie, Carole, and anyone who even came into view. I was all cutting and tearing edges and points. As before, with total acceptance of these irrational feelings, they drifted away as suddenly as they appeared.

By this time I was getting used to allowing any and all irrational feelings which came to me. I had been long conditioned to deny my feelings, especially if I could see no reason for their existence, i.e., if they were irrational. Tanya said to me that she believes that **all** feelings are irrational. Our rational thought originates in the neocortex and the origin of our feelings is the limbic system which is a few million years older than the cortex. Physiologically then, Tanya is correct. All feelings are irrational and only those which correlate with some immediate outside influence can have sense made of them by the cortex, the rational part of our brain. So this set of feelings is labeled 'rational' and the rest 'irrational.' The labels are inaccurate. Feelings are **sorted** by the neocortex into those it correlates with external events and those it cannot correlate.

To me, and I think to Carole, the only way to explain an irrational response in a healthy person is that it is a residue of a forgotten or repressed past-time matrix of events. When I meditate, random "irrational" **thoughts** drift into my mind. I have learned not attempt to will them to stop appearing. I simply look at them, acknowledge them, and let them drift away just as they drifted in. Now, for the first time, I see **feelings** as being similar to thoughts in this regard. They drift into my consciousness and, upon being accepted and acknowledged, simply drift away as do my random thoughts.[54] This is a whole new way of responding to my feelings. Thank you, Carole and Tribe, for teaching this.

---

[54] Paster, Marion, ibid, page 119:

"If we accept that the nature of feelings is that they move through us, then everything we feel can be fresh and new all the time. If we try to hold on to what we are feeling in one situation, the feelings appropriate to another time and another situation cannot arise."

Next came Vic. This talented man played church and theater organ wonderfully but he had more than his share of hang-ups and one of then was operating. Carole lay on top of him, with Charlie and me along his two sides, and we all began to fuse/pressure him. With Vic, I again became the father and son simultaneously but this time on a level that seemed more real to me. It began with an irrational feeling that entered my consciousness: hostility toward Vic. I accepted this feeling, just because, and my whole body quivered with rage at him. Why I felt this I knew not. About that time Vic began to moan and speak of great pain. It is hard to sort out what went on with others without their verbal feedback. I will simply describe what I **thought** went on with them here (which may be judgmental on my part):

To me, Vic's problem was the same, generically, as mine: sexual attraction toward mamma clouded over with guilt feelings. The difference was that Vic had not allowed his irrational feelings to consciousness so they still ran him. He was stuck. Perhaps his guilt was more firmly entrenched than mine. His guilt seemed to be combined with something else which I saw as dishonesty about his feelings. He continued to 'con' himself that his feelings did not exist while stuffing them deeper into his toe. It felt like he had a self-deceptive feedback mechanism—the one thing which will eventually blow anybody out of reality. My irrational anger toward Vic, which seemed connected to his pain, was the goading he needed to move through his block. With my hostile feelings acted out in fantasy, and with Vic's resulting groans, Vic began to move. I was acting on a higher authority that I could not understand: **the irrational** which was (today) my psychic father. My irrational father fed me just the right feelings needed to induce Vic, my surrogate son, to move through the psychic pressure that I laid on him by my act of welcoming my

irrational feeling about him. Again, there were three: my
son, me, and my father. We fused and flowed, in
equilibrium, with no boundaries. We had reached the
Triplepoint of the father/self/son relationship.

An image came to me: Vic, unclothed, stood on top of a
hill which was covered with broken bottles and jagged
glass. He seemed to say, "This is what I have to go
through and if you make me do this you will be hurting me
physically." This ruse, this excuse to avoid moving
through feeling, just enraged me. I felt this was a neurotic
defense against motion and Vic was trying to slip us into a
reality level where we were all committed to not physically
hurting anyone. That is, his fantasy image appealed to my
commitment to non-violence in the **physical** world as if he
could convince me that it applied to my **fantasy** world. He
didn't convince me that we were relating in the physical
domain where our common commitment to nonviolence
applied. This was subterfuge and it made me angry. In my
rage I responded by, in fantasy, rolling naked Vic down
that hill and shredding his psychic body with all that glass
he created. Just as I did this Vic uttered his loudest moan
yet and told me what pain he felt. I replied, silently, "If
you pull that kind of con job, man, I will call your bluff
and you will have to feel the result." Then I told Vic to
accept his pain, feel it with every cell. Then, at last, I felt
motion.[55]

After a brief moment, after he stopped fighting it, he
replied that the pain had vanished. He finally got to his
feelings and then to peace and **good** feelings.

---

[55] Here, I believe I was doing what Carole does when she "follows her
intuition" during a session.

Debbie then came over, hung up. I felt the same irrational feelings for the same purpose as with Vic: to motivate movement on her part. Carole was now off with another human pile. Debbie was surrounded by Charlie, Vic, and me. We all seemed to be in the same emotional space. Whether one approached sex energy or just plain good, warm closeness, we were blocked from these feelings by guilt. This common theme was what we worked with at that time, learning to allow these "forbidden" feelings into full awareness.

At this time I felt stoned out of my gills but never before had I remained completely tuned in on reality levels while so boosted. My unconscious was flowing like a river after a heavy rain and at the same time I was well tuned in on the operational activities in the room. For example, when Carole changed the music I saw her look down inquisitively and I responded with a hand signal about how loud the music was. Later, as Charlie and I spoke briefly about Debbie, I saw Carole signal with her hand to shut the hell up (her face was covered) and I picked this up and relayed her message to Charlie who was turned away from her. It felt absolutely wonderful to operate well on both inner and outer levels simultaneously. It had never happened before.

Down the road a little, Don had me on top of him with various people on top of **me**. Across the room Carole was on Debbie, Don's wife, working her through something. My task was to carry Don through to good feelings. As Debbie (who was being worked on) made noises of distress, I felt Don's psyche making tremulous efforts to go to her aid. Don, I felt, was too much under Tribe authority to squirt out much on the psychic level. Nevertheless, I felt that my job was to keep his psyche contained as Debbie, verbally, called out. In my imagination, I had the white sheet we were lying on picked up and draped over Don. Then I created an imaginary hammer and nails and nailed the sheet down to the floor all around Don at the edges. Every time I felt a quiver out of Don I would just imagine pounding another nail into a loose corner of the containing sheet and he would quiet down.

Twice I felt irrational hostility float into awareness and I responded by imagining tearing Don's body apart. The third time this happened I expressed it verbally. I told Don that I felt him being ice cold from the pelvis down and that he was avoiding his commitment to accepting good feelings and I felt pissed. After he acknowledged the truth of that he began to warm up.

One of the irrational feelings that came to me was that of feeling inadequate, totally inadequate. Given my particular dynamics, I think that is the most unbearable of all my feelings. Thankfully, it left as soon as I accepted and wallowed in it. As I pondered these events I saw a pattern emerge from allowing a few irrational feelings to **be** and watching the result in the person I was with. Then the concept of the irrational took on a new meaning for me and connected with the idea of being under valid authority, however irrational it appears. I was beginning to understand something about the irrational! With this realization I felt a warm wave of feeling adequate wash over me. Yummy! Hey, how did that **rational** feeling get in here? Who is guarding the door?

The session's aftermath was great fun. Quentin and I sold each other heaven and hell, Jane looked wonderful and floating. Carole looked exhausted but seemed to feel good. Her input was that she was proud of me—as I was of myself. I felt that I hadn't made such strides of growth and learning for many, many sessions.

$\mathcal{A}$ $\mathcal{B}$rush with $\mathcal{P}$sychosis[*]
Strange events of 6-8-67

I hardly know where to begin with this but last night was
when things began to get goofy. I got home from the
Thursday Tribe meeting reasonably early. Feeling like I
wanted to get some things done, I filled out a couple of
employment application forms. I was a bit groggy from a
hard day and from three glasses of wine I drank at the
meeting so I took 5 milligrams of methedrine at about 9:30
PM. Finding, then, that I really didn't feel like working, I
began to read a copy of a *Product Design* magazine while
waiting for the methedrine to impact me. Then I did a
crazy thing. I poured a glass of brandy and drank it even
knowing, from experience, that this stuff puts me out.
Thirty minutes later, nearly out, I went to bed. At about
2:00 AM I awakened, from the methedrine probably. I
couldn't sleep. Having had no sex in any form for several
days I began to masturbate. This didn't feel particularly
good and it took an hour or more before I came. Still
feeling agitated, I got up and put on some music. Feeling
like I wanted some wine, I examined the appropriateness of
doing so at this strange time of day. I thought it OK if I
committed to get up and be at work on time in the
morning, so I drank a glass or two hoping it would put me
back to sleep.

I arrived at work two minutes late but didn't feel this was
significantly off. At about that time I began to feel strange,
which I attributed to lack of sufficient rest and to a
hangover from the wine and brandy.

My draftsman had not arrived. He was the only other person working in my office and he was frequently late. I had trouble calling him on this because of my own guilt. After all, I reasoned, who am I to call my subordinate on coming in late when I, also, did this?

Then I lied. I signed on the board as "Am at engineering library," and headed for the cafeteria for coffee and some food. I hoped this would help me get going. Following this I stopped by the barber shop and got a haircut, still on "company time." I was feeling better by then but still not my normal, energetic self. I next went to the gym to shower off the uncomfortable hair clippings around my neck. The sauna in the next room was appealing so I went there for a while, hoping I could sweat out the hangover. It being too early in the day for others to come into the sauna, I compulsively began to masturbate. By then it was clear to me that something in my unconscious was operating. I realized that, since I didn't shower before leaving home that morning, I must have unconsciously planned all this beforehand. I finally got back to the office at 9:30 and began to do some work. Off and on I felt, again, strange. The radio was on and I listened to some news about the Middle East war. I thought I was picking up and carrying anxiety about it. At about 10:00, still feeling a lack of drive, I took another five milligrams of methedrine. I had resisted taking any earlier because I felt I had misused it the night before. At about 10:30 I took a "coffee break," so back to the cafeteria. There I noticed a woman I had seen there for the past two days at that time of morning. I felt extremely attracted to her; her beautiful face and body turned me on. I wanted to get to know her. Then I realized that I had unconsciously timed my coffee break to put me in the cafeteria at the time I thought she would be there. I decided that, next time I saw her, I would ask her if I could join her at her table and start a conversation. I couldn't tell whether she was a student or employee; she dressed more formally than a student (high heels, etc.) but she seemed to study a lot. I returned to my office and more work.

At 11:30 I began to work on my extracurricular project—my strobelight manual. I felt some guilt about doing this on University time but I pushed these feelings back into unconsciousness. Lunch went by quickly as I didn't have much appetite because of the methedrine I had taken two hours earlier. Having another thirty minutes of "lunch hour" I worked on my car radio but this work ran about twenty minutes into my afternoon work schedule. Walking back to the office I felt extremely strange, especially crossing a street. I felt myself at two levels of reality: one wanted to be careful crossing the busy street so as not to be hit by a vehicle, and the other was a vision of charging blindly across and being hit.

Back at the office I decided I would feel better if I did something constructive for my employer, the Physics Department. Successfully assembling a project in the shop, I took another coffee break at about 2:30. Intuitively I felt that the attractive woman would be in the cafeteria at that time and, yes, she was there. She was sitting with three people who looked like professors. I finished quickly and left, deciding to return in one hour and see if she was still there. Returning to my office I stopped by the post office to check my mail. This was where I customarily received orders for copies of my strobelight manual.[56] There was no mail. Leaving the post office I felt strongly hit by the strangeness. I felt my sanity was leaving me. It became hard to function, to navigate my way through space.

---

[56] The *Strobelight Manual* was a moonlighting effort of mine. This was a small how-to book I self-published and sold through classified ads placed in various underground newspapers.

Looking around for something to ground me I saw a water fountain and took a long drink. Things tasted and smelled most strange to me. I felt myself going psychotic. I wondered if someone had slipped about two hundred micrograms of LSD into the coffee I had earlier. I felt that if I allowed myself to go into insanity I would become violent and destructive and I would finally explode. I got to the street level of the post office building and went outside and headed toward the Physics building. I felt worse and worse. I felt like I wanted to put my hands into soil and carry some back with me. Instead, I walked up to a shrub and tore off a leaf with each hand, symbols of life and nature. They helped me somehow. I feared I would meet someone who knew me and I would be incoherent. Finally, after what seemed like a long, long walk, I made it back to my office. I sat down and pondered for a couple of minutes. I knew I needed help and I needed it quickly. I was operational enough to find Carole's number and began to dial her at home. I hung up and re-dialed her office number. I left my name and number with her answering service and waited for her return call. Putting my computer to work on this, I looked around and felt guilt seep into consciousness; I had not been doing the work I was paid to do. I sought out something to do that would be productive for the Department. Considering my state, this wasn't easy. The guilt leveled off but did not diminish. I took out paper and began to make notes on my experience.

The first thing I wrote down was the name of the Physics professor who had shot and killed himself elsewhere in the building six weeks prior. We had been close, he and I, and he had a long history of deep depressions. I felt he had been guilt-ridden. Not liking the look of his name on the paper, I erased it. I next wrote, "Why is death preferred to insanity?" I thought I must be close to the state the professor had been in when he killed himself. I didn't know why but I felt he killed himself to avoid going insane.

The emotional impact of my experience was so intense that I am convinced that, without my training and understanding of psychic manifestations gained in Tribe, I would never have made it back to my office. I had felt on the very edge of sanity.

Finally, I examined my guilt feeling. I realized that I had been dishonest with the Department in doing my projects on their time. I wrote down everything I could think of that I had done to contribute to my guilt. Not until I allowed my guilt feelings to consciousness did the load of insanity lift. I began to understand the cause and effect of my experience. I went through harrowing and terrible feelings as I examined all my dishonest acts of the past few weeks, as I realized how I had been pushing limits, everywhere, as far as I could. I became fearful of facing blasts from Carole and Tribe for this.

The more guilt feelings I allowed to consciousness the more the threat of insanity lifted.

Commentary
"What's wrong with this picture?" I remember these words from a childhood magazine showing a busy drawing containing several illogically placed items. Applying the question to my experience this day I had to answer, "Almost everything!"

    1) I had created a lot of guilt-feeling residue over the previous weeks;

    2) I had pushed the guilt feelings into unconsciousness, denying their existence;

    3) I had misused both Methedrine and alcohol **in combination;**

    4) I had convinced myself that I only had to

show up for work. In fact that was
necessary but not sufficient;
   5) When I got there I spent the work hours
on my personal projects, one after another.

The process of creating and accumulating my guilt feelings
combined with my conscious denial of them allowed them
to grow like a snowball rolling downhill. This could only
lead to an overwhelming breaking point at some time which
I could not, of course, see coming.

The leaves I held in my hands, which enabled me to return
to the relatively safe space of my office, remind me of
stories written by anthropologist Carlos Castaneda. On
more than one critical occasion don Juan, his teacher, had
Carlos rub handfuls of certain leaves over his skin. What
kind of grounding or psychic stability can one get from
rubbing vegetative matter on the skin? This is worthy of
investigation. Perhaps we might someday have a new,
topically applied, pharmaceutical product to control
psychosis?

A Vivid Apparition
9-21-67

Last night I saw an apparition. I fell asleep with the reading lamp on but turned very low—with the intensity of a night light. It was not bright enough to disturb my sleep but light enough to see most of the room clearly with my dark-adapted eyes. It felt to be around four AM. In a light sleep, and dreaming, I thought I heard a woman's voice in the room—one syllable—which woke me up. Lying on my left side, I opened my eyes and saw a figure standing beside me. The figure was facing toward my feet and so I saw its right side, in profile. It was wearing something that looked like a bathrobe which was dark green covered with small red squares. Its legs were occupying the same space as the bed but appeared to be standing on the floor. I didn't look down at the legs, however, as I stared at the face to see who it was. At first I thought it to be Carole, then it looked like Quentin, and thirdly it looked like Bob. It was not as if the face changed but that, in the dim light, my perception of it kept changing.

The persistence of this image stunned me. Not infrequently I had, in the past, gotten brief glimpses of apparitions which would vanish instantly the moment I focused on them; not so this time. This figure remained in my vision for ten to fifteen seconds. It appeared to adjust its sleeve and seemed to be talking with someone else. I did a double take on it at first because I thought I was still dreaming. My immediate reaction was to check this possibility out by looking around the surroundings—my bedroom. Nothing appeared out of place so I looked back at the form which was still there. If the light had not been on I knew I could have not seen anything in the room. I saw this figure with reflected light only; no local luminescence or ghost-like light came from it. I felt no fear at this presence but I believe I certainly would have had I not been knowledgeable and experienced with psychic phenomenon.

This is the only time in my life that such a thing has happened, and I have no idea of the meaning of it.

Acceptance of Brother
Tribe LSD of 10-21-67

During stash-dump Carole spoke, at length, about the
neurotic acting out of her husband Charlie the last week.
We collectively decided that he should spend the day
upstairs and not be part of the session. We each agreed not
to carry his load during the session.

Vic and I were paired for the session. I felt him clinging
like ivy on me. I felt hostility toward him for this grasping
thing which didn't seem to belong to the session. My
computer worked on this—how to deal with it so as not to
deflect from the overall issue of the day. I felt that we
should both be moving toward something
external—something beyond us both—and instead he had
been zeroing in on me. I had him lie on top of me but
with him facing upward instead of toward me. This forced
him to face toward something that was outside us both.
That worked. Then I was able to share, verbally, with Vic
what had gone on within me. His acknowledgement—that
he had been wanting to cling to me—confirmed my
intuitive insight. At this point something broke with us and
I no longer felt the alienation about him which I felt earlier.

This was interrupted by a fire drill[57] after which we both got to work in earnest and continued to do so for the remainder of the session. (At the end we were both drenched in sweat.) This is the first time in my life that my computer kept working **all** the time and without distracting me or deflecting the work at hand. I felt well integrated all during the day. Upon receiving inputs—information, feelings, imagery, etc.—I checked them out simultaneously on all levels: feeling, computer and sensory. The meaning that came from this went into storage until needed. The issues of **narcissism** and the **acceptance of brother** (our focus for this session) kept zooming into the day for me. I had done much work on these issues previously and had mistakenly thought them complete for me—but there they were. To accept the reality of **brother** I had to give up myself as the center of the universe. The issue kept swirling in my psyche. It looked all too much like what Charlie was supposed to have been working on upstairs and which we had been ordered not to carry for him. I don't think that I carried any of Charlie's load but it looked like we were all so intermeshed that we cannot help coming up with the same issue as the order of the day.

I visualized the idea of coming to terms with brother by seeing Israel and Egypt dynamically interacting. Egypt, apparently, did not like coming to terms with her neighbor one damned bit. Similarly, I saw the USA and USSR working out the acceptance of each other. By *brother* I mean that which symbolizes anyone on the other side of narcissism. If one or the other of USA and USSR "kills"

---

[57] The occasional "fire drill" was one of our safeguards. During a fire drill we simulated what we would do in the event that somebody knocked at the door during a Group drug session. We were prepared to assume a "normal" appearance. This was in keeping with our need to maintain a low profile.

then the whole world goes down the tubes so **that** solution to the narcissism problem is self-defeating. Just in the middle of my internal wandering through Russia someone played *The Great Gate at Kiev* from *Pictures at an Exhibition*. I laughed and wondered how many others in the room were in Russia at that moment.

Vic and I alternated as to who was on top. Lying face to face now, I felt our bodies fuse and flow together. To me, we felt like Siamese twins with our torsoes joined together by stitches running down our sides. Our organs were floating around and we shared some of them. With Vic on the bottom, Carole came and lay on top of me. For a few minutes I seemed to breath for Vic while his heart seemed to beat for me. Had we not been prepared, I think this fusing could not have happened. The preparation, strangely enough, consisted of learning the boundaries of our own bodies and psyches which we had been doing over the years in Tribe.

Pondering about the idea of bodily and psychic connections and boundaries, I was reminded of something Carole pointed out about litter a few times in the past. It was that the things with which we litter the countryside are really extensions of ourselves and if improperly disposed of there remains a thread of some kind connecting the litter to us. I thought of how careful I had become to properly dispose of my trash, since then, and how much less entangled I have felt as a result.

It felt vitally important that Vic and I hold together while fused and not let anything "leak in or out." It felt that, fused as we were, we had elected to relinquish the unique identity or ownership of our organs, blood, etc. In this condition—being unable to tell what belonged to me and what belonged to Vic—it felt critical that some stray book or ashtray not be allowed to drift into our space since it would have become incorporated into our bodies. This possibility felt potentially destructive. Also, if our mutual boundary opened for a moment a liver or kidney might float out and get lost. Where would we be later if that happened and we then separated? Besides, that would make a horrible mess on Carole's carpet.

I felt that all the hard work with my framework, over the years, had manifested itself in my skeletal system. Always before it felt like I had to hold myself intact with my muscles. This time I felt my rib cage supporting Vic's weight instead of sheer muscle power. It was much easier this time. The growth of bone is slow but steady and my work was paying off for me.

Fused as we were, Vic and I became a space ship and we buzzed around and through galaxies. Inside, we were pressurized and every once in a while some trapped air between our chests would bubble out with a farting noise as it blasted out through the pool of our mutual sweat. This, I thought, was overpressure in our space ship venting into the void surrounding us.

During the session I was being worked on by entities of some kind. They were sorting out my nervous system, uncrossing wires for me. They worked like telephone repairmen. I could feel tiny probes poking around my brain. In response to this probing I could feel muscles around my body twitching as certain nerves were touched. The entities used this method to identify which nerve was touched by watching which muscle twitched in response. Later I was called upon to help correct things in other people or entities. This was the first time that I was given the authority to do any of this and I was very pleased with it. I had learned certain areas of discrimination and this was the key to my ability to sort out malfunctioning in others. Mostly it was my unconscious that moved out and into the others I was helping, so I can't speak of specific activities here.

Every fifteen minutes or so Vic and I would look at each other and decide we needed a breather from the intense work we were doing. In the middle of the day I looked at my fingertips and they were all wrinkled as if they had been immersed in water. This is the third Tribe session this has happened to me. This time they were, indeed, immersed in water—in the form of sweat. I came to the conclusion that work sessions can be fun.

The Pain of Divorce
Essay of 7-28-68

Today, Sunday, was my big weekly visitation day with
Thea. My five visiting hours with her were most difficult
for me, emotionally. I rode it out well but did not become
fully aware of the what and why of events until after I
returned her to Tammy and went home. I felt extremely
tired and decided to drift into a couple hours of sleep. I
lay on the bed and relaxed my body and melted into my
fatigue. Then things began to drift into my field of view
like wood shavings which were being moved, one at a time,
from one pile to another. The newly created pile was right
in front of me where I could see the shavings and stir them
with my hands until a pattern that I could see began to
emerge. The pattern was a picture of my composite set of
perceptions with Tammy and Thea today, and my responses
were woven into this pattern as well.

Tammy had delivered Thea to my house for her visit. Thea
had been crying. Tammy had explained that Thea had just
been spanked for swearing. She looked at Thea and said,
"Adults have the prerogative to swear, but children do not."
This felt strange to me; I don't like double standards. The
only thing I could think to ask Tammy was who was
present when Thea had done the swearing. My problem
was that I didn't know what question to ask. Tammy left
and I asked Thea what words she said that were swearing.
She said she couldn't say them because saying them was
swearing at someone. I said that just telling me what the
words were was OK and not the same thing as swearing at

a person. She accepted this and said that her words were
"Damned bloody window." She explained that she had
been trying to open the small, side, wind-wing window on
Tammy's car and it was stuck and Tammy would not help
her with it. I explained to Thea that some adults did not
like to hear swearing and would get angry about it and that
other adults are not bothered by it at all.

So I lay there, expecting to drift into sleep, and all these
bits and pieces floated into view and I shuffled them
around into a meaningful pattern and as I did so I began to
feel very angry toward Tammy.

The realization came to me that " . . . *damned bloody this"*
and ". . . *damned bloody that"* was Tammy's personal
idiom and no one else in Thea's world used this phrase.
For Tammy to spank Thea for repeating that which Tammy
taught her, by example, filled me with a sense of outrage at
how Tammy was treating Thea. My worst fear since
Tammy began her struggle to have a child with me was
realized. We produced this offspring in the midst of a relationship full of strife. I had held out on having a child
because I believed that neither Tammy nor I was emotionally mature enough to do justice with raising children.

Now here Tammy was, punishing her four-year-old child
for emulating her mother. My God, if Thea is punished for
emulating her mother, then who on Earth can she use as a
role model?

Tammy, of course, had been under a lot of pressure what
with the strain of the divorce, etc., but for her to treat Thea
this way made me furious. I had lost custody of Thea and
there was nothing I could do to prevent more of this. I
found this realization most painful and, instead of sleeping,
I found myself sobbing in pain for Thea. I felt her life
experience must be miserable and there was nothing I could
now do to alter that fact. It felt horrible.

Thea was a beautiful and bright child. I loved her deeply and, during her brief five years of life, I felt great pain that she had to suffer such agonizing strife between her parents. This was exactly what I had feared would happen. Thea, who was clearly an extraordinary person, was born into an environment of emotional turbulence and she cemented nothing between Tammy and me.

By the time Thea was four years old Tammy and I were no longer living together. We were in such conflict that Carole and Tribe moved Thea into the household of Don, Debbie and their five children. Of course this seemed best for Thea, for she needed a stable family environment. The arrangement was that I would periodically come over and spend time with Thea. Also, once a week I would visit and share dinner with the family. Tammy had her own arrangement with them. After this I never again lived with Thea, who was so dear to me; I only "visited" her. This is what came of surrendering my will to Tammy, Carole, and Tribe. I trusted to them that this outcome, which I had feared might come to pass, would not happen and still it did happen.

While Carole believed that I had feared a re-creation of losing my child following her birth, ironically, my acquiescence to the will of these people was, indeed, a re-creation of my earlier experience with Terisa! In that case, when we learned that Terisa was unexpectedly pregnant—knowing that we were not ready for this—we decided to have the child adopted out. Succumbing to the intense emotional pressure brought down on us by my parents and other family members, we capitulated to them and canceled our adoption plans. On that occasion, also, it was tears that made me change my mind in the end. They poured from the eyes of my brother-in-law as he begged Terisa and me to keep our child, insisting we were making a horrible mistake and that we would make excellent parents.

So, losing Tammy and Thea was, for me, the **second** time in my life I lost my family—only this time psychotherapy was supposed to prevent it! Carole assured me that I would not lose this, my second child and yet I did.

It must have been deeply embarrassing to Carole. We had come to her to get our marriage fixed and at that she failed. She told me my wires were crossed and assured me that having a child with Tammy would be a wonderful experience for both of us. It turned out to be a multiple tragedy for us instead. Please Carole, don't do me any more favors.

In all fairness, Carole's efforts to harmonize our marriage were heroic. She kept us together for seven years which was probably about five years longer than we would have had otherwise. Still, were I in her position, I would feel like a failure where Tammy, Thea, and I were concerned.

Creative Dissociation
Ritalin Session of 11-22-68

I didn't ask anyone to attend and support me at this session until after it had begun—procrastination again! I felt apprehensive as I approached the session—felt something would have to be faced but couldn't get any information about what it was. Some indications had come from Carole: To get Tammy out of my system and possibly to get insight into Nancy's death.[58] I felt glad when Bob drove me in for my Ritalin® shot and then on to Carole's house where my friends were waiting for me.

People began working on my body as I lay on the massage table. They discovered, and worked on, assorted lumps in my gut. Carole said I was stuck on my hostility toward females; I responded by blasting, with her permission, Freda, who was the nearest attractive woman. As I did so the nature of the hostility came to me. I felt anger that came out in the shape of a ribbon, and it twisted ninety degrees from its source. It was the product of psychological dependency and, more specifically, sexual dependency. This insight came to me rapidly because Carole chose the right person for me to blast. Freda had

---

[58] This is a reference to the unexpected death of a female Group member. Nancy was a creative and troubled artist. She had succumbed to a deadly combination of alcohol and Seconal®. Her death was officially listed as a "possible suicide." Just how or why Carole thought we could possibly derive insight into her death from my session baffles me to this day.

felt the most open, warm and sexually flowing to me as I hugged everyone when I first entered the room. This enabled me to see the connection between my hostility and my sexual dependency almost immediately. With my hostility discharged, Carole had me lie down again and the body work continued. In specific parts of my gut I felt great pain. Quentin said he felt my muscles defending and said I should open up. I had no trouble feeling this in my body also.

My struggle here was to do three things simultaneously: 1) loosen up my muscles, 2) keep the pain in my consciousness, and 3), scream my anger. These tasks felt mutually exclusive to me. In order to yell I had to tighten up my abdominal muscles. But I was to keep these muscles relaxed! Quickly I discovered that the only way to achieve this was to squeeze out my screams with the upper part of my lung cavity by somehow pulling my ribs in toward each other. The resulting yells came out more like grunts than blood-curdling screams but they were effective and my emotions kept flowing. Very slowly, I allowed the pain to surface and loosened my gut. I was learning the art of **creative dissociation**. The pain level was terrible and I went through—and to completion of—something indescribable.

This concept of creative dissociation was crystallizing out as a technique I was learning in Tribe. This was ongoing and not something learned in a flash of inspiration. It is a useful means of body control I occasionally use.

The most memorable occasion was years later when I crushed the tip of my thumb, up to the first joint, in an industrial accident. The pulp that used to be my thumb had to receive seventeen stitches without anesthetic for it once more to be a useful thumb. Using creative dissociation I was able to keep my right arm, hand and thumb totally motionless for the doctor as he sewed it up. The pain of the needle was too intense for my body not to tighten up. What I was able to do was choose which part of my body would respond to the needle, and I successfully kept the muscular response confined to my **left** arm.

This technique has been an essential part of my learning to relax and I think it should be taught with relaxation training. In the dentist's chair, I used to sit with my hands trying to crush the armrests with my lock-grip. Once I learned to set my mind to scanning my body for tight muscles to loosen, instead of keeping my consciousness in my mouth . . . once I learned to keep my consciousness from concentrating at the tooth being drilled, but instead keep it diffused throughout my entire body, I could keep my body relaxed. Under these conditions, pain did not dominate my consciousness and from then on I stopped needing and requesting novocaine.

I flipped over and eyeballed with Carole—my hands on her shoulders. Having just swallowed some water I had a gas bubble which would not rise. This bubble became part of the drama. It harmonized with the process of discharging junk from my body. It felt like a constriction in my throat; it made it difficult to push other bubbles, water, vomit, junk out. I pushed and pushed—and little by little it came up and out. I was screaming at Carole as I pushed out with my diaphragm. Carole was gripping my neck and I felt the sensation of having the venous blood flow shut off to my brain. It reminded me of my childhood. I must have been anemic or something because when my blood sugar dropped I would nearly faint if I stood up suddenly. As I screamed at Carole with her hands on my neck I blacked out momentarily. I felt that, during this brief moment, something in my unconscious made an important change. Some learning fell into place; Carole taught me something and I don't yet know, consciously, what that was about.

The scene of yelling, relaxing and opening to pain was a three-way, simultaneous event which could not be complete until I had learned to capture all three at the same time. This was the monumental task for me. Any one of the three, by itself, or even any pair, was not difficult. It seemed to take forever for me to get all three together. However, the moment I **did** get all three simultaneously Carole said, "It broke," and I reached another Triplepoint in my life.

The neurosis can keep control with one or two things at a time but not when I got all three going. I saw it, in imagery, similar to the pea and three walnut shell game. The element "pain" could be put under the shell labeled "masochism" or under one called "motivation-to-evolve," for example. As long as there was an empty shell, i.e., I wasn't experiencing one of the three, there was an empty space into which the neurosis could move. This left another empty space behind it so more motion, more slippery cleverness, could follow. This could go on endlessly until I existentially achieved all three: yell, relax, and allow pain; no empty spaces for the first time. At that moment all three shells became occupied and the neurosis froze. The three items stopped shifting, stopped changing labels.

It felt like doing all three at the same time should be called "creative dissociation." Yet, another perspective is that I was simply learning to be an integrated person with the resulting complex internal organization. I was learning to allow many simultaneous feelings and experiences including allowing the feeling of fear of the abyss. . . fear of being overwhelmed. The learning came from realizing that I don't have to become overwhelmed as I had believed. My capacity to live was being expanded as I overcame my fear by opening my consciousness to it.

During my lunch hours at the University I had been either swimming a quarter mile or playing a couple of games of handball. My body felt like it was singing. Surely my resulting excellent physical energy level was necessary for this session's work. The sheet draping the massage table on which I lay was wet from sweat. Brothers and Sisters, you who assisted me at this flowing and productive session, thank you for your love and energy.

Do I Still Belong Here?

Dream of 6-3-70 (about five months before my termination from therapy.)

*I arrived at my house and there were many Tribe people
there, like at a party. I entered and saw that the interior had
been completely changed. The furniture, pictures, etc., which
I had there had been, for the most part, changed for other
items. These new things had a different style and feeling.
There was a dining room set, chairs and table, which seemed
similar to Carole's but not her specific set. They were from
the same period of ornate carving in dark hardwood and with
plush seats. In my closet many boxes of my junk (i.e. things I
hang on to but never seem to use) had been cleared out.
Tribe children were there who were playing with a litter of
very young Siamese kittens.*

*I didn't know what had happened to cause this change and I
became furious that it had happened.* **Who** *had the nerve to
enter my life and make such changes without checking with
me! I felt angry but didn't know who did this. I felt that it
must have been a Tribe decision. I also felt specific hostility
toward Yana and Doris, two of the lesbian Tribe people,
because they had been staying at my place and I felt they had
a significant part in the changes. I went to Carole (for whom
I also felt hostility since she probably had a hand in it) to get
information. I did have enough objectivity* (how is one
objective in a dream?) *to keep the hostile feelings in check
until I learned more about this since it was based only on the
interpretations which I had made. I found Carole upside
down standing on her head. She was physically straining,
doing one of her exercises. I asked her about these changes*

*in my home and she replied in a very vague fashion and not
at all like her real response would have been. It was as if my
question took her completely by surprise and she said something like: "It seemed to us that you had died." At about this
time I awoke.*

It was then about five months until my resignation from
Carole's therapy. My unconscious was losing its enthusiasm for this particular growth process and was
beginning to rumble of encroachment.

A Revealing Encounter

Tanya, my friend of many years, had been in Carole's therapy and Tribe for only about two months, corresponding to my final two months in this environment. Since she came into Tribe through me, I think she was, in the end, perceived, by Carole, to be too aligned with me—and therefore too dangerous—to keep around. So, a week after I left, Carole kicked Tanya out also.

Being in this unusual environment for such a short time, Tanya did not have much exposure to the Tribe paradigm. She had not learned much of what was expected Tribe-member behavior. Earlier, Tanya had had considerable Gestalt therapy and she had progressed into serving as leader of Gestalt groups, for two years, for the Harvard extension program. She wasn't naive about group therapy, only about Carole's version of it.

Shortly prior to my last "Power Session" there occurred a Tribe meeting that neither Tanya nor I shall ever forget. Tanya and Carole were standing in Carole's living room facing off one another. Carole was interrogating Tanya about some now forgotten context. Others in the room were scattered around, both sitting and standing; most were focused upon this confrontation. Carole became highly irritated at Tanya and eventually slapped her, hard, on the cheek, as she was wont to do with recalcitrant patients. Tanya had never seen Carole slap anyone and didn't know the routine. She said, calmly, "Oh, so that's how the game is played . . . OK," and then slapped Carole right back, on **her** cheek.

At the instant of the slap I happened to be watching Paula who, herself, was watching Tanya and Carole. Paula's eyes got big and round, she drew in her breath sharply, her mouth fell wide open, and her hand went up to her throat. To all appearances, she couldn't believe what she had just witnessed. To her, and others in the room, Tanya had done the unthinkable.

Upon being herself slapped, Carole shouted, "Grab her, she's violent!" Tanya was then immediately held, arms and shoulders, by those who had been standing behind her. Carole then let loose with a verbal tirade about how invalid Tanya was. Among other things, she accused Tanya of killing her son who, at the age of four, had run in front of a passing car. According to Carole, this past event had been engineered by Tanya's unconscious "deadly hostility[*]." This accusation was not an isolated event; over the years, I had seen Carole make similar accusations of having "deadly hostility" to others in Tribe who were unfortunate enough to have suffered a similar loss.

Here we have two adult women. One slaps the other. When the other returns the slap, the first accuses her of "violence." Clearly there are two standards of behavior here. During my years in Tribe I had readily accepted this double standard. After all, we, the sick ones, had come to Carole, the healer, to get well; of course she knew best. Now, decades later, I find such a double standard absolutely absurd. Arguably, a slap on the face may have some therapeutic shock value, but it is always a demeaning experience for the patient, and it clearly displays a lack of respect for his or her autonomy and integrity.

Most of Tribe had been immersed in Carole's therapy for so long that the double behavior standard was little questioned or even very visible to us. We went into shock upon witnessing Tanya return Carole's slap. Watching the wide disparity between the responses of Tanya (to Carole's slap) and of Paula (to Tanya's slap) was, to me, revealing. It showed me just how encapsulated I had become in Carole's way of doing things; that realization shocked me a second time during this event. Carole's therapeutic modalities, which once I had admired in their originality and daringness, now appeared somehow **encrusted** to me.

Omega Box: My Final LSD Session
10-28-71

In fall of 1971 I was called in to Patrick's 'Power Session' during the afternoon to do body work on him. As I massaged his back Carole looked at me and said, "You need one of these." I didn't feel especially warm toward the idea but said nothing. Later, I scheduled my own 'power session' with her for late October, 1971. I knew that if I didn't Carole would have challenged my resistance. How different this attitude was from my early years of therapy when I, instead of Carole, initiated the sessions out of a felt need. Here is my report for this session, which I wrote a full year after the event. This, of the scores I have written, is the only one I did not submit to Carole. I wrote it for my own sense of completion.

Report of Power Session[*]

There is no way to go back. . . What you left there is lost forever; at a time like that what's important to all of us is the fact that everything we love or hate or wish for has been left behind.
— Carlos Castaneda, *Journey To Ixtlan.*

It took a whole year to begin to fully understand what happened that day in October. Early during the session I had vivid imagery of, among other things, a cage with bars, which I called **Omega Box.** It was cubical in shape, suspended in space and just large enough to hold one person. It was similar in shape and size to **Alpha Box,** the "glass box" I had imaged during one of my very first LSD

sessions twelve years earlier. The difference was that this
had confining bars instead of protective glass for sides.
The similarity of these boxes, at beginning and end of my
tenure in therapy, is reflected by the chapter titles; *alpha*
and *omega* are, of course, the first and last letters of the
greek alphabet. The imagery was accompanied by feelings
of fear of being locked up in a cage. I didn't verbalize this
to anyone. I asked myself, on the computer level, what did
it mean? I took it very literally: I was afraid of being put
in jail and the only way to have that happen was to be
arrested and the only thing in my life which was illegal was
possessing a small amount of marijuana.

I thought my unconscious was giving me warning that my
lifestyle was in danger because of this one exposure that I
had created. So, quite simply, I decided to stop the only
illegal practice in my life and silently committed to myself
to do this. I thought—should I tell this to Carole? I pondered the idea for thirty minutes and called her over and
started to tell her. Before I could finish this she interrupted
me and started a chain of questions and answers that took
us to a place unexpected by me and which ultimately led to
my being sent away. I had, you see, admitted to directly
violating a Tribe Rule and had been doing so for some
time. Carole said, "This boggles my mind, I'm going to
get Charlie" During the intensive inquisition I underwent
by Carole, Charlie, and later Chuck and Carlos, I found
myself almost detached in a way. Chuck and Carlos were
Carole's beefy teenage sons and both had powerful
personalities. I was, however, neither in their emotional
space nor was I in the space they thought I was. I
contributed to this situation by deliberately exaggerating
historical facts about me. I didn't want a repeat of the time
I made it with a woman at Cambridge, which was
destructive to my marriage, and they, at a Tribe meeting,
had to drag the facts, kicking and screaming, out of me

through my resistance. So this time I went to the other extreme and gave them "an extra measure of the facts." Some part of me was totally fascinated with what was happening.

This event took place a year ago. A few days ago my unconscious led me to re-read all the material I have in my file labeled: 'Tribe stuff since last Power Session', including all the notes and correspondence. Reading about the imagery of the cage I was struck by a totally different interpretation. I saw the cage and the fear it invoked to mean that my life—at that time—was already nearly as locked up as if I were caged. Carole had been telling me what profession to enter: Rolfing, even though I had told her twice I didn't want to do that. She told me what people to spend my time with and where to go for vacations and with whom. She told me with whom to have sex and with whom to live. I could go on and on.[59] My life was very unsatisfactory to me and the situation was getting worse instead of better. Tribe was my emotional family and Tribe life had many rewards but it also had many sources of conflict. Conflict will always be with us but I was beginning to wish I could **choose** some of the things which brought me to conflict. That is why I felt fascinated by watching the process of my falling out, even being expelled from therapy and Tribe. At the time I had no inkling that Carole feared me and what that fear was

---

[59] H. Strean and L. Freeman, "Confessions of a Psychoanalyst" *New Age Journal*, May/June 88:

"...an axiom of psychoanalysis: Never tell a patient how to live. The patient has a right to self-determination. ...I am absolutely convinced people feel their best and function best when they decide for themselves what will make them happy. When rules, regulations, or modes of behavior are imposed on men and women, they resent the rules, fight them, and feel like small dependent children who are expected to ape and echo their parents."

making her do, and that was a large part of why I could not understand what was happening.

Meanwhile, back at my Power Session, my unconscious—under the influence of LSD—was trying to tell me something. My conscious mind felt in a state of naive innocence; I didn't get the message. For example, I had a flash of imagery early in the day of a doctor holding a person's wrist. The act was ostensibly to take the pulse of the patient. The imagery shifted. The doctor began to squeeze the wrist in a terribly tight grip and a look of hatred appeared on his face. Under cover of appearing to heal, this doctor was actually trying to squeeze the life out of the patient. I didn't know what to make of this imagery. Some time later in the day Carole sat on the bed beside me and took my wrist in her hand in exactly the same way as in the first part of my earlier imagery. I thought—at the time—that seeing her do this simply reminded me of my imagery and I blurted out a description of it without any thought. I think that Carole must have, on some level, thought I was referring to her with all my talk of invalid doctors during the day.

The reason I felt detached during the intense questioning was that I was not emotionally where people thought I was and where they were telling me I was. Charlie kept repeating, "The magnitude of what he has done hasn't hit him." Carole had asked me—in reference to my smoking pot without her permission thereby breaking a Tribe rule, "What did you do with the guilt?" Her presumption—that I would be overflowing with guilt—was not accurate. However, I felt that if I told her I felt no guilt that she would slap me "back to reality," as she sometimes did with her patients. I knew her mind was made up about the existence of my guilt and, rather than deny it I gave her an answer I knew she could accept even as I knew it to be untrue: "I masturbate the guilt away." This only

contributed to her already inaccurate picture of my inner
state but by then I was intrigued with the way things were
unraveling. I began to see the possibility of getting
disconnected from the forces that were almost totally
controlling my life[60]. In fact, I had thought that I **did**
have her permission to smoke pot and therefore I felt no
guilt because of that.

In some ways I think Carole was her own worst enemy.
Her attitude of arrogance and all-knowingness made her
vulnerable to a distorted model of reality. Because she has
such certainty, she is not open to alternatives and, sometimes, to asking the right questions. Years earlier, when I
faced the threat of getting fired from my job, I sought
Carole's assistance. She helped me compose a letter to my
supervisor which ". . will give him reasons he will understand." I kept the job and learned from the experience.
Now, during my questioning, I was giving Carole,
". . reasons she could understand."

Following my 'Power Session' I stayed the night at
Carole's house as was customary so I would not drive with
any drug left in my body. As I was about to leave, the
following morning, Carole told me that I probably would
not understand the reasons for what she told me to do but
that I was to do these things anyway, as if I did understand.
I didn't know it at the time but what happened between
Carole and me, between Tribe and me, and between Carole
and Tribe were **all different things**. There was no open
communication between these relationship entities. Carole
must have thought I had become aware of her Achilles'
heel. At the time, I wasn't aware that she even had one,

---

[60] Extricating oneself from Carole's Tribe was a problem. In my ten years
with it I never witnessed anyone leave with Carole's blessing although she assures
me that many did and I have no reason to doubt her.

but her fearful behavior actually led me to it eleven days later. Just what this behavior was I'll get to later.

During this session I got under Carole's skin in more than one way, although this was neither deliberate nor was I conscious of doing so at the time. I spoke disparagingly of "invalid doctors" and named a few of the series of M.D.'s who had provided her with medical coverage only to leave her later in an atmosphere of strife. I never suggested that I felt that Carole, herself, was an invalid doctor but, somehow, this idea was in the air.

During the afternoon, Mary came into the session. She was a beautiful single woman and we shared a mutual attraction. While Carole was out of the room, I propositioned her to have sex with me there and then, on Carole's bed. Mary, responding to my grossly inappropriate proposal, backed off and said, "I'm going to get the boss." Carole came in and we discussed this. Carole was visibly upset. I was goading her, but consciousness of that fact didn't come until later. A week or so previous to this I had asked Mary for a date and Carole, overhearing this, wedged into the conversation and got herself included on this date. I think she wanted to prevent any strong bond forming between Mary and me. We three spent a pleasant evening at Mary's house. Then Carole and I left together and I gave her a ride to her car, which she had parked near my house. Now I believe Carole left her car near my place to insure that I did not spend the night with Mary. By then it was past eleven PM. Carole seemed to be expecting or hoping that I would invite her to come home with me. She had left Mary's with a tall cocktail in her hand. I walked her to her car and she got in. I said goodnight to her and walked away. I left her sitting behind her steering wheel, still holding the cocktail.

At my Power Session I didn't know how Carole felt about my requesting sex with Mary on Carole's bed, as she didn't comment about her feelings. Later, however, I was in the room by myself for a while. Having to pee I entered the bathroom. Returning to the bed I heard a sound through the open second story window. I looked out and saw Carole punching the blazes out of her heavy punching bag down below. I later described this scene to Bob (who had lived with Carole for a while and knew her habits.) He showed astonishment and said that he had never seen her do that during a Power Session.

Termination from Therapy and Tribe

The Thursday following my Power Session, November 2, 1971, Carole instructed me to get a prescription for chlorpromazine, (a so-called "chemical straight jacket"), a **big** prescription. "You are going to need them," she said. She must have called Dr. Adams's office to clear this because when I arrived there I was handed a bottle of one hundred and twenty caps! I had never taken chlorpromazine before but I knew what they looked like, and I had never seen anywhere near that many in one place.[61]

Carole also told me: "You must act **as if** what I have told you is true and do what I tell you because you probably won't feel it on your gut level." Of course I consented to this. After all, when one surrenders power to a therapist one must trust what she says regardless. She said that I am cut off from my feelings and so won't feel the truth of her utterances. In cases like this the patient can only trust in the intact integrity of the therapist. I later concluded Carole's integrity had **not** been intact—in this instance—and that she was sacrificing me to cover her own LSD trail.

During my final regular (Thursday) Tribe meeting, five days following my final Power Session, Carole had called

---

[61] At this writing, eighteen years later, I still have one hundred and nineteen of them. I once took one of them out of curiosity to see what kind of experience chlorpromazine produced. I was very nearly physically and emotionally unable to function; for someone as active as I, it was terrible.

in most of the Monday Tribe members in addition to the usual Thursday bunch; her large living room was quite crowded. She devoted the entire evening to "Trevor's problem," conducting a character assassination on me the likes of which I have never witnessed before or since. She started with a long monologue about how serious this problem with me was, how far out of reality I was and how I had dumped everybody with the monstrous thing which I had done to myself, to her and to tribe. She emphasized how near to "going crazy" I was. She held me responsible for a mouth lesion that had shown up on innocent Sarah's dental x-ray. This was because I had been in relationship with Sarah and had invalidly impacted my oral tissue by smoking pot. Therefore, Sarah was "carrying my load." Then Carole passed the chair around the circle and **everyone present** stood up in turn and proceeded to tell all how sick, invalid, and dangerous I was. It was like a baton of evil discourse, created by Carole, being passed around from person to person. My only response to each of them was to look in their eyes as they spoke their piece. I absorbed all they had to say in total attention and in total silence. This seemed to take hours but I wasn't watching the time. Afterward Carole billed me thirty dollars for that tribe "therapy" meeting.[62] Incredibly, I survived the evening and got back home intact. I attribute that to my incredible strength of character gained from Carole's years of rigorous therapy.

---

[62] Actually, her bill for this 'service' arrived many months after I left. Before I resigned from therapy I had paid Carole's last bill for my final Power Session and Carole thanked me, in writing, for "payment in full." Almost a year later, she wrote me that the person who had been doing her billing had failed to bill me for my final Wednesday Group meeting and Carole had just discovered the fact. After all that, Carole requested belated payment which I refused.

A few days later, under orders, I left Bridgeport and drove to Catskill with $3.68 in my pocket. I left without being able to obtain homeowner's liability insurance to cover me when someone rented my home. I moved in with Tanya and began the search for a job working "in the wilderness" as a logger's assistant, as I had been instructed to do.

At the following Tribe meeting, November 9, 1971, (attended by Tanya but not by me) Carole questioned Tanya about me during the mid-meeting break:
"If he starts to talk crazy give him a Chlorpromazine."
Tanya, in response:
"What do you mean by 'talk crazy'?"
Carole:
"If he starts to discuss me."

After the break the meeting continued. Carole questioned Tanya:
"What is Trevor's attitude?"
"He doesn't want to be cut off from Tribe. He didn't feel guilty because he was telling himself he had permission to use pot. He now acknowledges that wasn't true, but since he has told the truth he is now clear (back in integrity) and he feels he should be accepted and helped to complete this matter."

At this Carole inexplicably got furious with her and yelled, "She's protecting him!" and ordered her out of the house. Tanya started toward the door and was stopped, physically, by several of the Tribe members who refused to let her leave, saying, "Don't you dare leave." Tanya stood and asked, "What will it be, go or stay?" Carole screamed at Tanya, "Get out of my house!" and to Tribe, "Let her go!" The Tribe did so and she left.

Tanya was puzzled by this push-me pull-you situation. Being a relatively new member of Tribe, she did not know that many times in the past a patient—in fear, anger or frustration—had attempted to leave a Tribe meeting and been prevented from doing so. Carole would always yell to the Tribe, "Don't let her go in that condition! She will hurt herself driving home." At this, Tribe people physically restrained the person, preventing her from leaving until the issue at hand could be carried to completion and the person could be at peace with it. This had become routine and Tribe was conditioned to always restrain the person. Carole's demand that Tanya get out of her house was contrary to this conditioning and, to Tribe members, contrary to safe therapy. This was unprecedented behavior on Carole's part and it must have puzzled many in Tribe. I wonder how Carole explained it to them after Tanya left?

Tanya drove back to Catskill and joined me. She gave me a rundown of the evening's events. When she told me that Carole had instructed her to give me Chlorpromazine if I started talking about her I finally had the critical missing piece: I knew then that Carole was, for some reason, afraid of me. I had only to search my memory for what she might be afraid of and I quickly realized what it could only have been: at the start of my Power Session Carole had given me two Sansert® pills (structurally related to lysergic acid butanolamide[63]), a glass of water, and a tiny white square of paper which I recognized as "blotter acid", also known as ashless laboratory filter paper on to which a precise amount of LSD-25 had been deposited by pipette. She said to me, "For my other patients I have to shred the paper and mix the LSD in with the water so they won't

---

[63]   Sansert is a prescription drug sold for treatment of vascular headache. It inhibits the effects of serotonin and is reported to induce mild LSD-like hallucinations, when ingested in quantity, as a side effect. Any hallucinations reported by Carole's patient may therefore be attributed to the Sansert. Earlier Carole used another drug, Romilar®, a commercial cough syrup, for the same purpose.

know what they are getting, but, with you, I don't have to do that." She didn't bother to conceal the LSD because I had a long, reliable and trustworthy track record with her. Why did she volunteer this information to me? I think that she wanted me to know others were not treated so openly and that I should be discreet when talking with them. Subsequent to those statements, during the middle of my Power Session I told Carole that I had been doing something that was in violation of a Tribe rule: smoking marijuana without her permission.

So Carole had given me compromising information and afterward I gave her reason not to trust me. By then, however, it was too late; she couldn't remove from my memory what she had told me earlier. I had become a loose cannon to her and she must have feared I would tell Tribe members that she had been giving them LSD without their knowledge.

Carole's fear was groundless for two reasons:
 1) I would never have released her secret; in spite of how she felt about me, I **was** trustworthy and,
 2) Tribe people already knew what they were being given during Power Sessions (they weren't stupid); it just wasn't openly talked about, that's all.

Not knowing these things, however, Carole had only one recourse and that was to isolate me—seal me off—from the rest of Tribe. She attempted to do this on all fronts. At first I was to go far away and work outdoors in the wilderness. Later that was changed and I was to move to Catskill and live with Tanya. I was not to return to Stamford for "some months." I was not to communicate with anyone in Tribe except Henry. I was to ingest Chlorpromazine®. I was described to all the Tribe as "about to go crazy," hence anything I might be heard to say could be attributed to a deranged mind. Carole instructed everyone except Henry to avoid **any** communication with me. Tanya's description of her final Thursday Tribe meeting (November 9, 1971) gave me a new awareness of what was motivating Carole. I examined the rest of the pieces and they all fell into place. I now understood the maelstrom I had been riding: the Chlorpromazine, the isolation, the order to communicate with only Henry, and all the rest. It suddenly made sense to me. Realizing that the part about my "going crazy" was spurious I felt immensely relieved. When you are outnumbered by thirty or forty trustworthy people who are unanimous in their opinion that you are going crazy, it will leave you shaky, however untrue their collective opinion may be.

Earlier, when I did speak with Henry, I had told him I had additional information for the Tribe. What I had wanted to convey was that I had deliberately exaggerated my description of violating Tribe rules. Carole, I guess, thought the additional information was something different though, and she immediately sealed me off from Henry and had me communicate with Quentin instead. Quentin told me that this change had been done because "Henry was getting 'entangled' with me."

As for the massive guilt which Carole expected me to have for smoking pot without her permission: I had asked for, and received, permission from her to smoke many times during the previous year. Each time I requested her clearance she responded with the question: "Does it help you?" Upon replying yes to this, and insuring the circumstances were safe, she always consented to my request. Since this question was always asked, I eventually decided to smoke pot one evening without asking for her clearance. Hell, I knew what question would be asked and I could ask it as well as she. So, rather than take up her time with getting permission I simply took over her role as questioner. That didn't make it legitimate but I convinced myself that it did.

Later Carole (inadvertently?) reinforced my position: Late one evening I got stoned and Carole happened to telephone me. I answered and after hearing my voice she said, "It sounds like you are into something . . . give me a call tomorrow, would you?" Then she disconnected. She had sounded friendly and warm. I took this to mean that she, in her superior perception, had realized that I had been stoned and that was OK with her.[64] So, from then on, I felt no hesitation in checking myself out instead of having Carole check me before I smoked pot. By the time of my November Power Session when I 'confessed' to her that I had been smoking pot without her permission, I was really twisting what I saw as the truth. I truly believed that I **did** have her permission but set that aside and described to her the situation but omitted this belief. I manipulated this subtle point during the Power Session to see what the outcome would be. Later, when I wanted to submit this missing piece, that is to 'fess up to my lie of omission, I was not allowed to. This explanation is not to defend my action but to describe why I did not have the guilt Carole assumed I must have had. Beginning with this false premise she followed a path to an incorrect conclusion.

Finally, with my new understanding of these events—gained from Tanya's new inputs one week later—I felt free to write my letter of resignation from therapy (and from Tribe as well, since it was impossible to be in Tribe without also being in individual therapy with Carole):

---

[64] Carole wrote me a letter in Spring of 1962 in which she described a telephone conversation with another patient. As soon as she heard his voice she accused him of being on some kind of drug which he indignantly denied. To her, his denial was clearly a lie. This is only one, of many, reasons I had for believing that Carole could read her patient's minds, even over the telephone.

Dear Dr. Govren,   11-12-71
     At our last meeting, on Nov. 2, 1971, you in-
formed me that there was a strong likelihood that I
would "go crazy." You then ordered me to leave
town, leaving behind my home, my friends, and my
means of livelihood, for an indefinite period of
time, forbidden to communicate with you either by
telephone or by mail.
     From this I find the conclusion inescapable that
you neither have my best interests in mind as your
patient nor are you operating with the high professional standards which I had expected.
     Therefore, it is my desire to conclude our
relationship at this time.

Sincerely, signature

In Carole's reply letter she stated that the process of going
crazy had, evidently, already started. I have never doubted
that Carole had read these two letters to Tribe. After a
week of deep thought, I wrote her another letter:

Dear Carole,   11-20-71
     You have badly misjudged me in many ways, one of
which being on destructiveness. I have no desire
to harm you or your professional reputation (although I suppose I should, considering what you
have done to mine). My principle feeling toward
you now is one of gratitude for twelve years of
excellent service rendered me.
     You have taken precautions to prevent me from
leaking certain information to the Tribe. I assure
you it is quite unnecessary, and in the process a
lot of innocent people are being trampled. One
person who needs and wants your help has been
kicked out of Tribe as a result. Also most or all

of the Tribe are in more pain than necessary because you have transformed me, overnight, into some
kind of lethal, destructive, monster. I expect
that this latter thing is also causing you some
problems in the credibility gap dept. So please,
for everyone's sake, call off your wolves.

By the way, if my information is correct, at the
point in time when you were passing Catskill and
felt "malevolent forces" I had not yet left Bridgeport.[65]

Yours, signature

To this letter Carole never responded and I don't doubt that
she did **not** read this one to Tribe. Eighteen years have
elapsed since these letters were written. During that
interval Carole lost, first a patient, and then her license to
practice. The information revealed in this book could no
longer threaten her career. The night after I wrote this
letter I had a dream:

---

[65] I was informed that Carole stated to Group that as she was driving past
Catskill—at a time she believed me to be there—she had felt "malevolent forces"
coming from there, presumably emanating from my presence.

A Disturbing Dream
11-21-71

*I was in a large office building where I worked. In came
Carole, Charlie and Dick. I gave Carole something to
read. She went over to a large display island on the floor
similar to ones in department stores to display goods.
There she read what I had written and it had a devastating
effect on her. She got so angry and furious that her blood
pressure rose until something happened—a stroke? Several
people went over to her to attend to her needs only to
discover that she was dead. Her body was lying atop the
merchandise island. Charlie looked at me knowingly and
said, "I know what is at the bottom of this", meaning that
he knew that I was responsible for killing her. He began a
flurry of activity trying to gather evidence that I had done
Carole in, going through papers and things. He started
into one of the nearby offices and I said to him, "Get out
of that office." He stopped, turned around, and looked at
me but he didn't leave the doorway to the office in which
he stood. I was feeling huge anger and felt very powerful.
I began to move aggressively toward him and he left the
office. Later I learned that he had filed a legal suit against
me for the sum of two million dollars. I didn't feel particularly worried by the lawsuit but felt it as a kind of
irritation.*

This dream occurred shortly after I left therapy. It is laced
with both magic (words that kill) and paranoia (gathering
evidence to support a belief that I used my magic to kill.)
My unconscious seemed to concur with my notion of why I
was expelled from Tribe.

Carole's Conflict

All through my years of therapy with Carole she was faced with a conflict of interests. This was not her fault; it was the fault of our medical delivery system. Doctors in the United States are generally paid when you are sick and not when you are well. This applies to clinical psychotherapists as well as to physicians. So when a patient left Carole she received one fewer paycheck every month. In my life experience I have noticed that there is a direct correlation between the competence of therapists and their freedom to release a patient. Their feeling of inner security is a function of their competence at healing people and hence their ability to replace old, released patients with new ones who want, also, to be healed.

Early in my years of therapy with Carole she occasionally mentioned the event of release of her patients to "go their own way." In the latter half of my experience with her, however, I don't remember her mentioning this at all. Once in a while a patient would announce, at regular weekly Tribe meeting, that she or he felt ready to leave therapy. Carole's reply seemed sincere, warm and open. She would say to her patient, "It is wonderful that you feel that way, however you still have an unresolved problem in the "X" area of your life. Why don't you stay until this last problem is worked out and then leave?" Whereupon the patient would stay . . . and stay . . . and stay. Both the problem area and the request to leave would become buried in subsequent events.

Dr. Jay Haley writes about the hypnotherapy of Milton Erickson:[66]

Erickson does not seem concerned about the patient becoming overdependent upon him. . . he manages to begin termination with the moment of contact and future disengagement is part of the intensity of the relationship established. Because of his positive view and his respect for patients, Erickson is willing to start a change and then release the patient to let the change develop further. He does not allow the needs of the treatment setting to perpetuate the patient's distress, as can happen in long term therapy. Since he does not see therapy as a total clearance, or cure, of all the patient's present and future problems, he is willing to give the patients up.

When I terminated from Carole's therapy and from Tribe I did so under a very large, grey cloud. I was unanimously made wrong by all. Had I, at that time, read the book: *When to Say Goodbye to Your Therapist* by Catherine Johnson, Ph.D.[67], my load would have been much lighter following my closing this chapter of my life. Mainly, I would have learned from it that what had happened to me also happens to many, many others as well.

Dramatic passages from Johnson's book that reverberated in my soul out of my own therapy experience are:

---

[66] *Advanced Techniques of Hypnosis and Therapy;* Selected Papers of Milton H. Erickson, M.D., ed. by Jay Haley, page 541.

[67] Simon & Schuster,
Simon & Schuster Building,
Rockefeller Center
1230 Avenue of the Americas
New York, NY 10020

page 11: When leaving is entirely the patient's idea, as frequently it is, a therapist may throw up roadblocks. You are not "ready," he may say, implying that your desire to terminate reveals a wish to run away from your problems.

page 12: You thought you were better and suddenly you are hearing from your therapist that you are not—worse, that your desire to leave therapy is a sign that you **need** therapy. Abruptly you see your newfound self-reliance metamorphosing into just another symptom. Faced with a resistant therapist, you must either rebel and declare yourself cured—a process that can be painful indeed—or sink back into business as usual.

page 49: If you have changed in all or some of the ways you hoped to when you entered therapy, you are right to leave—**even if by staying you might go further yet.** In therapy, there is no such thing as "all the way." You can always be in therapy; you can always find something new to talk about, or something old that threatens to live and breath once more. There is no shining moment when suddenly your life becomes fail-safe, when suddenly you are fixed and happy and whole for the first time.

page 76: When a therapist believes that normalcy does not exist (except as a reassuring fiction), he will automatically look for the "dark side" and hidden conflicts in anyone who appears actually to be normal. This means that no matter how much progress you make, your therapist is still going to perceive remaining conflicts and potentially dangerous problems.

pages 195-6: . . . in trying to decide whether or not you are involved in a power struggle of whatever dimension, you should look for even the subtlest signs that your therapist is trying to hold you in a dependant role. After all, the proper goal of therapy is to help you achieve **independence.** If your therapist ever so slightly puts down your accomplishments, or ever so slightly but consistently casts doubt on all your major relationships, these innuendoes will tend to make you feel that you can't go it alone- that now is not the time to leave.

Reading these passages was a déja vu experience for me; I had already been there.

Is There Life After Tribe?

When I made my break, even after piecing together what had really taken place, it was important to me to make a complete and total transformation in my life.

I relocated to the heart of silicon electronics development, Concord, several hundred miles distant. My new occupation was something that had always been an anathema to me: I became a **salesman.** My new "family," the firm that hired me, wanted me to peddle a subsidiary product line they had acquired: electronic equipment for the behavioral sciences. My new abode was an apartment instead of a house. Everyone I related with, professionally and socially, was new to me. I moved from a situation with incredible social support, Tribe, into one where I had to start from scratch from ground zero. None of my new co-workers knew anything about psychotherapy or my history with it. To them, I was a "normal" employee with whom to work and sometimes play. What they saw in me was what I brought to them. For a long time I scrutinized their responses to me to detect any perception they might have that I was in any way insane. I carried this insecurity with me for several months before I felt secure that the conditioning I received upon my expulsion from therapy had been spurious. As a salesman I drove a brand-new luxury car; this had never been my style. I became part of the daily ritual of The Company sales crew: the lavish lunch together at one of the several nearby posh restaurants.

My style had been to brown-bag lunch inside the laboratory with my fellow engineers.

So you can see the extent to which I turned my life upside-down and inside-out. I force-fed myself as much **change** as I could manage. I needed to fit myself into something where I was valued by people and I almost immediately achieved that. My career working at University laboratories gave me almost unique experience interfacing with both electronic data gathering equipment and the research professors who used such hardware. The people at my new work place welcomed me with open arms. After all, I was a competent professional who could accomplish desired things for them. I served them for about two years. In a strange sense this was a period of penance for me. I opened myself to experiences never before considered such as playing the role of salesman.

Finally I followed a path I had been drawn toward ever since I discovered the wilderness during my childhood. In Summer of 1974 I drove to the west coast and searched around Southern Oregon and Northern California for "my country place." I found it in September and escrow closed the following month. As I struggle to support a life, now without the possibility of a regular paycheck, I remain in contact with a several other ex-Tribe members. To this day we remain warm friends.

My literary mentor, Carl Jung, offers an opinion[68] on the role of groups such as Carole's:

The secret society is an intermediary stage on the way to individuation. The individual is still relying on a collective organization to effect his differentiation for him; that is, he has not yet recognized that it is really the individual's task to differentiate himself from all the others and stand

---

[68] Jung, Carl, *Dreams, Memories, Reflections*, page 342.

on his own two feet. All collective identities, such as membership in organizations, support of "isms," and so on, interfere with the fulfillment of this task. Such collective identities are crutches for the lame, shields for the timid, herds for the lazy, nurseries for the irresponsible; but they are equally shelters for the poor and weak, a home port for the shipwrecked, the bosom of a family for orphans, a land of promise for the disillusioned vagrants and weary pilgrims, a herd and a safe fold for lost sheep, and a mother providing nourishment and growth. It would therefore be wrong to regard this intermediary stage as a trap; on the contrary, for a long time to come it will represent the only possible form of existence for the individual, who nowadays seems more than ever threatened by anonymity. Collective organization is still so essential today that many consider it, with some justification, to be the final goal; whereas to call for further steps along the road to autonomy appears like hubris, fantastically, or simply folly.

Nevertheless it may be that for sufficient reasons a man feels he must set out on his own feet along the road to wider realms. It may be that in all the garbs, shapes, forms, modes, and manners of life offered to him he does not find what is peculiarly necessary for him. He will go alone and be his own company. **He will serve as his own group**, consisting of a variety of opinions and tendencies- which need not necessarily be marching in the same direction.

The emphasis is my own. Although I didn't read this opinion until recently—it was unearthed in research for this book—it heartened me. This is my ultimate vindication for my decision to terminate from therapy. Both Carole and Carl Jung have impacted my life substantially and positively but, in the end, I must "write my own book."

The strange, only partly conscious, suspicion I had at the end of my Tribe tenure—that it was becoming unhealthy for me to linger in therapy—is also addressed by Dr. Jung: page 344: Anyone who attempts to do both, to adjust to his group and at the same time pursue his individual goal, becomes neurotic.

On the Meaning of Authority

The words *authority* and *author* come from the same root. There are three kinds of people: those who can write, those who can read (but not write), and the illiterate.

Many hundreds of years ago, when the only books were fully handcrafted by a few monks, there were very few readers and even fewer authors. Most of the populace could not read. Thus, a person who could not only read but also write was held in highest esteem. The author was authority. Now our society is saturated with printed matter. The root derivation of the word *authority* is not presently so obvious but is still retained in a few places. The program I use to write this book, Wordperfect®, has an organizational tool called *Table of Authorities*. It is used by lawyers who refer to written law to support their arguments. Many footnotes in this book refer to another author—as authority—in support of my arguments. I do this with full knowledge that other written works, by other authors, can probably be found to refute those from whom I quote. It is written that one can support almost any side of any argument by quoting the right piece of scripture, chapter and verse.

Until I entered psychotherapy I had never bothered to examine the meaning of *authority*. Like many words in my vocabulary I "learned its meaning" from the context in which I heard it used time after time. During the course of my psychotherapy my relationship with the concept of authority evolved in stages. The first thing Carole taught me regarding it is that there are two kinds of authority:

valid and invalid. This was, for me, a critical point; emergence and use of this key distinction transformed my life. Of course I had, in my past, often been subject to invalid authority and my reaction was to deny **all** authority as only quasi-valid. Sometimes it was valid, sometimes not. This very inconsistency gave me justification to feel indifferent toward all authority. Therein derived lots of problems for me. The results of not "rendering unto Caesar that which is Caesar's" caused me all manner of punishment and grief I might have avoided.

Once I began to discriminate between valid and invalid authority things changed for me. The immediate impact was that I had a tool for avoiding the repercussions of flouting valid authority by simply not flouting it. I learned how, as Carole put it, to be **under authority.**[*] Slowly, as I cleaned up my rebellious behavior, much of the stress I underwent vanished. Many people and institutions stopped demanding accountability from me; I was no longer giving them reasons to do so. I was under their authority. I began to pay my bills on time. People backed off. I began to have more time and energy to get on with things important to me where, before, I had felt yanked around.

My early image of authority was that it was absolute. Carole taught me that it is relative. One has authority based upon superior education or life-experience but always in a specific area. My doctor is an authority on my body's anatomy/physiology but not necessarily on anything else. The Boston traffic cop is a law enforcement authority in that, but not in any other, city.

With time and experience in making these discriminations there grew in me a kind of self-confidence. The opportunity to challenge invalid authority, once I stood on solid ground, became my option which replaced my prior self-defeating rebelliousness. I learned not to attempt to challenge authority unless 1), I knew what I was talking about (and could, if necessary, back up my position), and 2), I was willing to devote the non-trivial time and energy it would require.

A former FCC commissioner, Nicholas Johnson[69], offers a plan for challenging invalid authority which he calls "The law of effective reform." It is so empowering that I want to share it with you. Johnson writes:

In order to get relief from legal institutions (Congress, courts, agencies) one must assert, first, the factual basis for the grievance and the specific parties involved; second, the legal principle that indicates relief is due (constitutional provision, statute, regulation, court or agency decision); and third, the precise remedy sought (new legislation or regulations, license revocation, fines, or an order changing practices). When this principle is not understood, which is most of the time, the most legitimate public protests from thousands of citizens fall like drops of rain upon lonely and uncharted seas. But by understanding and using the right strategy the meekest among us can roll back the ocean.

Johnson then describes how **one lone person**, using the law of effective reform, removed all tobacco advertising from television! John Banzhaf, a young New York lawyer, wrote a letter to the authorities in Washington about a "fairness complaint." He pointed out that a CBS-owned television station (the specific party) ran a lot of cigarette commercials. Then he referred to a legal principle, the "fairness doctrine," which provides that a broadcaster has an obligation to present all sides of a controversial issue in its programming (the legal principle). The remedy he sought and achieved was for the FCC to order the TV station to present the omitted point of view regarding

---

[69] Johnson, Nicholas, *How to Talk Back to Your Television Set,* Bantam Books, 1970, page 188.

cigarettes: the health impact of smoking. Banzhaf won his case. Anti-smoking commercials began to appear on television. Rather than allow this truth to be presented to the public, the tobacco industry simply stopped television advertising totally.

As I learned, through experience, to relate to authority I began to assume my own authority based on my particular areas of expertise. In Tribe events, various roles of authority were discussed and set up. One person was chosen as ritual authority. Another was to be food authority. Another was assigned the authority to direct the Tribe activity at a given point in time. We practiced being in positions of authority and being under others who, themselves, were assigned roles of authority. We challenged each other's authority in these psychodrama-like roles. We learned how to discriminate between valid and invalid authority and we learned how to challenge invalid authority. These skills, among others learned from Carole and Tribe people, made me a very different person from the one who knocked on Carole's office door for the first time.

Personal Responsibility Is Personal Power

This is not about social responsibility which is what happens when you keep your agreements. This is about personal responsibility which is what happens when you decide to take total responsibility for your life experiences.

When a minor or major catastrophe befalls you what is your attitude about it? Suppose you are driving to a job interview and you get a flat tire on the road. This will make you late and soil your clothing and certainly impact your chances of being hired. What goes through your mind as you change your tire? Do you blame the tire manufacturer for making a defective tire? Do you blame the highway department for not picking up nails on the road? Do you blame yourself for going to a critical interview riding on bald tires? Do you blame yourself for not allowing extra contingency time to get to your interview?

The concept of blame is unproductive. It deals with what is past and therefore unchangeable. It holds yourself or another responsible for what has happened to you.

If you hold **yourself** responsible for an outcome then, next time around, you can arrange for a different outcome, one more to your liking. You can change your future happenings. If you hold **another** responsible for an outcome you have no way to change the outcome in the future. You do not have the ability to change or "fix" an institution or, in most cases, another person.

Personal power is the ability to make changes in future outcomes. You can induce change only in one person, yourself. Therefore, in order to change your future you must take total responsibility for your present. If the responsibility for what happens to you is laid on others then you have no chance of changing your future outcomes; you are powerless; you are, and will remain, a **victim** of those others whom you hold responsible.

When you realize that you create your own reality you can then begin to shape it. When you come down with a cold you might, for example, ask yourself:

Why did I create this? Perhaps I let my physical health run down. Perhaps I need to study more about how to keep up my level of resistance to disease. Perhaps I need to learn something about nutrition and my need for micro-nutrients, the forty or so chemicals my body needs every day which includes the vitamins, minerals, trace minerals, and amino acids.

It would be an excellent idea, I think, if each person were required to live by him or her self for a year or two prior to getting married. In doing so, experience would be gained in taking total responsibility for oneself. Then, when married, the partner would come into your world and lighten your load, by however much or little he or she did in the union. If you were brought up in a sheltered home you got, as I did, spoiled. There was, most always, someone who would cook for you and keep you intact. If you go directly from that lifestyle into a marriage you will never learn what it means to be responsible for everything in your life: your cooking, housekeeping, money management, transportation, health, and all the rest.

Without the experience of living alone you will expect your new mate to do all for you that your parents previously did. He or she will certainly not meet these expectations and, eventually, you will meet another reality which you will find difficult and puzzling. This is especially true if your new partner holds the same unrealistic expectations that you do.

Without the experience of living alone you will encounter disappointment that your needs are not being met. However if you enter a committed living-together relationship from a living-alone condition you will go from the freedom, independence, and exhaustion of being totally responsible for everything into a world which you share with someone else who will then pick up much of your load in life.

Dr. Paster's wonderful way with words[70] clarifies this issue.

page 48:
"Freedom entails responsibility, and the idea of responsibility is fearfully encumbered for most of us. In most families, "taking responsibility" for anything means to be guilty and at fault. Few parents demonstrate by their behavior that taking responsibility for oneself and for one's experience of the world is a fine and empowering way to live.

page 152:
"To take charge of our lives, we have to be willing to take responsibility for them.

page 154:
"...we've got to be willing to look at what we are still doing to keep ourselves in ... negative situations. If we are in a relationship or a job we don't like, we can start questioning, 'What are the choices I am making that are keeping me here?'

---

[70] Marion Paster, PhD, op. cit. For more on this contact:
The Institute for Personal Change
2295 Palou Ave.
San Francisco, CA 94124

Glossary

Akashic record	According to Cerminara, writing in Many Mansions, pps 44-45: "*Akasha* is a Sanskrit word that refers to the fundamental etheric substance of the universe, electro-spiritual in composition. Upon this *Akasha* there remains impressed an indelible record of every sound, light, movement, or thought since the beginning of the manifest universe. The *Akasha* registers impressions like a sensitive plate, and can almost be regarded as a huge candid-camera of the cosmos. The ability to read these vibratory records lies inherent within each of us, depending upon the sensitivity of our organization, and consists in attuning to the proper degree of consciousness much like tuning a radio to the proper wavelength."
Anima	An archetype of the collective and personal unconscious described by Carl Jung. A magical, feminine, mischievous being who changes into all sorts of shapes like a witch. She is both dreaded and adored by man.
Animus	As Anima is to man, Animus is to woman.

Aperture	An opening into a psychotic part of the collective unconscious to which the guilt-laden expose themselves.
	.
Authority, to be under	To have an attitude of compliance and respect toward some body of authority.
Asepsis	Contaminated by guilt or general malevolence.
Carbogen.	See page 111.
Cyanosis	The bluish color of the skin and mucous membranes due to reduced amounts of oxy-hemoglobin in the venous plexuses. ref: Medical Resident's Manual 2nd ed.Kennedy, et al. Translation: Blue skin is seen when there is insufficient oxygen being carried by the blood.
Exorcism	The process of expelling a foreign psychic entity from the body of its victim.
Hostility, deadly	Anger of such intensity that its carrier would like the object of its projection to die. The urge to kill. Carole, not infrequently, informed Tribe of the widespread existence of

"deadly hostility" in our world which we should be prepared to meet.

Hypnogogic imagery	Imagery occurring during the transition period between awake and asleep.
Infection, psychic	A state whereby one is being run by a pocket of ongoing psychopathy. One's appearance is subtly different in this state and this difference is discernable to the experienced eye.
Intuition	The pipeline to one's unconscious mind, our only input from life beyond our senses.
Karma	The East Indian philosophy of Karma yoga is based on liberation (or bondage) through positive (or negative) action; i.e., the yoga of action. The moral residue of one's acts does not go away, this philosophy says, but must be faced to completion if freedom from human bondage is ever to be achieved.
Load, psychic	An emotional or health burden one carries, on an unconscious level, for someone else. A wife, for example, gets a genuine headache thereby giving her and her husband a socially acceptable means to avoid attending a

party. She knows her husband does not wish to go but will not duck his duty on his own. She carries his load and "rescues" him with her headache.

Mescaline

The psycho-active ingredient of peyote, with psychedelic properties similar to LSD-25.

Methedrine®

A brand of methamphetamine or "speed".

Mummification

A therapeutic process one may undergo by either being wrapped in a sheet or being held, hand and foot, by a multiplicity of Tribe members. Sometimes this was accompanied by blockage of the subject's breathing passages. The containment was considered "complete" and was terminated when the subject psychically "moved." The event of one "moving" was ascertained by Carole either when her intuition detected the event or when the subject turned blue from cyanosis*, whichever came first. The rational for this was to deny **physical** movement thus forcing the desired **psychic** movement or psychic change.

Narcissism	An infantile state of fixation on one's self. When carried into adulthood it becomes psychopathological.
Neurotic	The state where one's reality-orientation is disturbed and he is in pain about it. Also the tendency to live in the past or future rather than the present.
Patient	Submissive victim. A detestable word used by the "medical delivery system" which keeps the people it serves from getting too uppity. Considering the disproportionate amount of wealth it sucks from society it is easy to understand why tactics like this are needed.
Psychotic	The state where ones reality-orientation is profoundly disturbed and he is indifferent about it.
Ritilan®	A brand of methylphenidate, a central nervous stimulant with properties similar to the amphetamines.
Shadow	An autonomous complex, made up of the negatives of the ego's positives. That which comes between a man and his fulfillment. Also the dark background from which we have evolved.

If you enjoyed reading

Triplepoint; LSD in Group Therapy, A Life Transformed

please let a friend know about it.

For additional copies use this order form:

- -

Please send me _____ copies of *Triplepoint.*

Base price is $19.95. Mail order terms are:

California residents: $24.40 tax and (domestic) shipping
included.

Out-of-state: $22.95 (domestic) shipping included.

Enclose check or money order, U.S. funds only.

Your
name_____

Address_____

City, State, Zip_____

Telephone_____
(In case of a problem with your order)

Send to:

Green Fir Publishing Company
598 Innovation Road
Petrolia, CA 95558

Errata sheet for *Triplepoint:*

1. Marion Pastor's name incorrectly spelled "Paster," pps 8, 210. My apologies, Marion.

2. Add to glossary:

Spansule®   A sustained-release form of drug packaging.

Tribe   The label which evolved for the collection of Carole's patients. Being heavily used in daily conversation *the Tribe* became truncated to *Tribe*. The word *Tribe* was used without the definite article *the* freely by its members. The word *Tribe* was spoken as a term of endearment by its members.

Unconscious, collective   According to Jung, ". . .part of the psyche which can be negatively distinguished from a personal unconscious by the fact that it does not, like the latter, owe its existence to personal experience and consequently is not a personal acquisition. It owes its existence exclusively to heredity."

A DISCLAIMER from Trevor Trueheart

Triplepoint is a *history* book. It describes events that took place in a different time and in a different social climate. This is a book about certain insights I attained during the course of psychotherapy administered by a board certified psychologist.

That this psychologist administered LSD—then classified as "experimental"—to some of her patients, under strict medical supervision as an adjunct to her therapy is true, but that is *not* what this book is about. This book is about the insights I attained in this therapy and how they helped me get well and grow emotionally; it is about transformation. Many of these learning experiences were so unusual and beneficial that I wrote them down so that I could share them with others.

Medically speaking, we cannot abuse drugs or substances; we *can* abuse our bodies and we *can* abuse our standing in society by advocating that others abuse their bodies whether with illicite drugs or by any other means.

With regard to illicite drugs, we currently live in a climate of fear. One store, so far, has rejected the book *Triplepoint* as a sales item based solely on the fact that the title contained the name of a drug that is now illicite. My book has been banned! Never mind that the described use of this drug (which was incidental to my psychotherapy) was, at the time, completely legal and socially sanctioned. In fact I then received (and still have) my doctor's prescription for LSD!

My consumption of LSD took place in a hospital room with both a medical doctor and my psychologist in attendance. Conditions could not have been more controlled than that and LSD was not, then, illicite.

I do not, either in my book or on this show, advocate illicite drug use. So-called "street drugs" are of unknown origin, unknown quantity, composed of unknown constituents, and were created by an unknown person whose sole motivation was greed. To ingest such material is, to me, nothing but stupid. In fact, if you read *Triplepoint*, you will learn why I think it stupid to flagrantly violate the law—any law—whether or not you feel it worthy of your respect.

That our society has chosen to respond to recreational drug use as a law enforcement problem instead of a medical problem is tragic. This mis-guided response has put our courts and criminal justice system into gridlock and we cannot build prisons fast enough. It has sucked our social resources away from education, health care, you name it. That LSD has the potential to heal and cannot, now, be responsibly used to do so, is equally tragic. I do not advocate illicite use of LSD. I do advocate changing the social climate so that, eventually, our legislators will once more place LSD into the hands of competent professional therapists where its benefits instead of its hazards will come forth. It is in this spirit that *Triplepoint* was written.